THE 12-SECOND SEQUENCE™ JOURNAL

Shrink Your Waist in 2 Weeks!

Jorge Cruise

Potter Style

Also by Jorge Cruise

The 12-Second Sequence™

The 12-Second Sequence™
(audiobook with audio trainer)

The 3-Hour Diet™

The 3-Hour Diet™ Cookbook

The 3-Hour Diet™ for Teens

The 3-Hour Diet™ On-the-Go

8 Minutes in the Morning®

8 Minutes in the Morning®:
Extra Easy Weight Loss

8 Minutes in the Morning®:
Flat Belly

8 Minutes in the Morning®:
Thinner Thighs and Hips

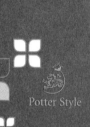

Potter Style

Copyright © 2007 by Platinum View Properties, L.P., a Nevada limited partnership.

All rights reserved.
Published in the United States by Clarkson Potter/Publishers, an imprint of the Crown Publishing Group, a division of Random House, Inc., New York.

Potter Style is a trademark and Potter and colophon are registered trademarks of Random House, Inc.

A companion to the book *The 12-Second Sequence™: Shrink Your Waist in 2 Weeks!*

by Jorge Cruise, with new material. *The 12-Second Sequence*™ was published by Crown Publishers, an imprint of the Crown Publishing Group, a division of Random House, Inc., New York.
www.clarksonpotter.com
www.crownpublishing.com
www.12second.com

ISBN 978-0-307-39556-6
Printed in the United States of America
Design by Danielle Deschenes

10 9 8 7 6 5 4 3 2 1
First Edition

FROM THE DESK OF JORGE CRUISE

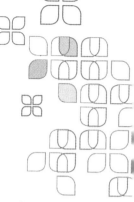

Dear Friend,

The 12-Second Sequence™ is a new way to exercise that will give you maximum results in the least amount of time. And it's all about shrinking your waist in two weeks! What's the secret? Well, as my good friend Dr. Mehmet Oz often stresses, it's all about muscle. You see, adding lean muscle tissue to your body is critical to weight loss because it's what drives your metabolism.

The problem with a lot of other strength-training programs is that they never allow your muscles to achieve maximum fatigue. Too often they focus solely on the quantity of the workout, and not the *quality* of the workout. The 12-Second Sequence™ focuses 100 percent on the *quality* of the exercises. By slowing down each exercise to a 10-second motion and

> **"Here's the big secret laid bare.** In the long run, you can't lose weight without building muscle, so follow Jorge's recommendations."
>
> —Dr. Mehmet Oz, author of *YOU: On a Diet*

2-second motionless hold, complete muscle fatigue is achieved and you add amazing, fat-burning muscle to your body faster and more effectively than ever before!

You will need to read my 12-Second Sequence™ book to get all the details, but in a nutshell, you just need to know that you'll be working out **only twice a week for 20 minutes.** You'll notice immediately that this plan is different than anything you've tried before. The very first week, even the very first day, you'll notice your muscles feeling more fatigued than after other programs. Your body will become more toned, more firm, and much sexier! Your clothes will fit better and everyone will notice how great you look. Moreover, you'll feel stronger, more fit, and see your waistline shrink within the first two weeks. Visit 12second.com for a free video class with me.

As a bonus to accelerate your results, there are two extra-credit items I will ask you to do: (1) eat right and (2) pre-breakfast cardio. What's the key to eating right? The first key will be to set your metabolism in motion throughout the day by eating every three hours. This is super important because it helps control your appetite and keeps your metabolism revved. You also need to make sure that you're eating the right amount of nutrients each day. On our plan you will eat a ratio of 40 percent protein, 40 percent carbs, and 20 percent fat, six out of the seven days. Then, one day each week you will get an optional "free-eating day." At 12second.com you'll find a video class on the eating plan and some fantastic recipe ideas.

What is pre-breakfast cardio? That is the other extra-credit item I recommend if you really want to accelerate your success. You see, in the morning before you "break" your nighttime fast you have a great opportunity to tap into body fat if you do a short, intense cardio session. Your body will be forced to burn fat for energy since you will not have eaten anything yet. During the 8-Week Challenge, I recommend getting in 20 minutes of morning cardio every day—it's quick and easy and will speed up your amazing results.

This journal is going to be crucial to your success with the 12-Second Sequence™. It's chock-full of inspiration and useful tips to keep you passionate about your goal. Read the daily meditations and take advantage of the success tips. Read the visualizations and really see yourself reaching your goals and succeeding at this program. Peruse the daily quotes and think of ways they apply to you. Write down your thoughts and feelings every day and reflect on them when you're feeling unmotivated. Jot down your reactions to the exercises and use those notes to help you in your next 8-Week Challenge. This journal is here to help you; take it with you everywhere you go.

So my challenge to you right now is to commit to this program 100 percent for the first two weeks! Turn to day 1 of this journal and get motivated to pick up your dumbbells and start the program today. I promise you will see your waist shrink dramatically and you will feel extraordinary. Then, continue the challenge for the remaining six weeks. Bottom line, at the end of the 8-Week Challenge you will look great in a bathing suit! I also want to invite you to join our free $100,000 Challenge for extra motivation. Visit 12second.com for details.

I look forward to seeing you online.

Your coach,

Jorge Cruise

TRACKING YOUR SUCCESS

On the following pages you will find a sample Eating Planner and two sample Workout Logs. Use these to guide you as you track your primary and secondary workouts and to help you stay committed to the eating plan. You can also visit 12second.com for a free downloadable 7-Day Grid, which allows you to monitor your eating and your workouts on one simple sheet.

You will also find a Success Contract, which will help you outline your reasons for doing this program and the goals you want to accomplish. You'll notice that the last line reads, "I Want to Feel." Use this to define how you want to feel at the end of the 8-Week Challenge. Do you want to feel strong? Confident? Fill out your Success Contract today and put it on your refrigerator—it will provide extra motivation for you every day!

The last way to track your progress is to use the 8-Week Workout Chart. Cross off each day as you make your way through the program. Whichever method you choose to track your progress, be sure to pick one you can stick with throughout the program.

EATING PLANNER (SAMPLE)

This plan will ensure leaner muscle and a higher metabolism.

Breakfast>time 7:30

Description

● PROTEIN* (3–5oz/40g)	smoked salmon
● CARBS (½ cup or 1 slice of bread)	whole-grain bread
● FRUIT (1 cup)	cantaloupe
● FAT (1 teaspoon)	1 tsp. flax oil on toast

Snack>time 10:30

Description

● WHEY PROTEIN SHAKE (1 scoop)	Jorge's Packs choc. shake

Jorge recommends Jorge's Packs™ protein drinks. > See other recommended snacks at the back of the journal.

Lunch>time 1:30

Description

● PROTEIN* (3–5oz/40g)	turkey burger
● CARBS (½ cup or 1 slice of bread)	whole-grain bun
● VEGGIES** (2 cups)	mixed greens
● FAT (1 teaspoon)	flax dressing

Snack>time 4:30

Description

● WHEY PROTEIN SHAKE (1 scoop)	Jorge's Packs vanilla shake

Dinner>time 7:30

Description

● PROTEIN* (3–5oz/40g)	chicken breast
● VEGGIES** (2–4 cups)	broccoli florets
● FAT (1 teaspoon)	olive oil

Snack>time 10:30

Description

● WHEY PROTEIN SHAKE (1 scoop)	Jorge's Packs choc. shake

*If you weigh under 150 pounds, eat 3 ounces of protein at every meal; if you weigh over 150 pounds, eat 5 ounces of protein.

**Veggies = nonstarchy vegetables.

Water (eight 8-oz cups) ● ● ● ● ● ● ● ○

Multivitamin ●

Primary Workout

DATE 1/7 DAY 1 OF 56

Start>time 7:00 Finish>time 7:20
TOTAL TIME 20 minutes

Select weights so that by the end of the fourth rep of each exercise you feel an intensity level of 8.

	Muscle Group	Exercise	Weight Used	Intensity Level
CIRCUIT 1	LEGS	beg. squat	N/A	6
	BACK	pullover on Swiss ball	5	8
	CHEST	incline on Swiss ball	10	8
	ABS	curl-up crunch	N/A	8

At this point you should be about 6 minutes into your workout.

	Muscle Group	Exercise	Weight Used	Intensity Level
CIRCUIT 2	LEGS	Swiss ball squat	N/A	7
	BACK	bent-over rows	10	8
	CHEST	push-up on knees	N/A	8
	ABS	chair crunch	N/A	8

At this point you should be about 14 minutes into your workout, including 2 minutes of transition time.

	Muscle Group	Exercise	Weight Used	Intensity Level
CIRCUIT 3	LEGS	plié squat	5	6
	BACK	hypertextension	N/A	8
	CHEST	flat dumb. fly	5	8
	ABS	broomstick twist	N/A	8

At this point in your workout you should be at 20 minutes. Congratulations! YOU DID IT!

BONUS CARDIO 26-MINUTE MORNING POWER WALK ●

After my workout I feel energized

(e.g., confident, strong)

WORKOUT LOG (SAMPLE)

Secondary Workout

DATE __1/10__ DAY __4__ OF 56

Start>time __7:30__ Finish>time __7:50__

TOTAL TIME __20 minutes__

Select weights so that by the end of the fourth rep of each exercise you feel an intensity level of 8.

	Muscle Group	Exercise	Weight Used	Intensity Level
CIRCUIT 1	SHOULDERS	standing shoulder press	10	8
	BICEPS	standing curl	10	8
	TRICEPS	chair dip	N/A	8
	ABS	toe reach	N/A	7

At this point you should be about 6 minutes into your workout.

	Muscle Group	Exercise	Weight Used	Intensity Level
CIRCUIT 2	SHOULDERS	standing lat. raise	10	8
	BICEPS	side curl on Swiss ball	10	8
	TRICEPS	dumb. skull crusher	5	7
	ABS	Swiss ball crunch	N/A	8

At this point you should be about 14 minutes into your workout, including 2 minutes of transition time.

	Muscle Group	Exercise	Weight Used	Intensity Level
CIRCUIT 3	SHOULDERS	seated rear delt raise	5	7
	BICEPS	preacher curl on ball	10	8
	TRICEPS	standing tri. kickback	10	8
	ABS	lying obl. twist	N/A	8

At this point in your workout you should be at 20 minutes. Congratulations! YOU DID IT!

BONUS CARDIO 26-MINUTE MORNING POWER WALK ●

After my workout I feel __motivated__

(e.g., confident, strong)

My 12-Second Sequence™

SUCCESS CONTRACT

Photocopy and place on the refrigerator, in the pantry, or at your bedside.

Today's date_____

> MY TWO-WEEK GOAL: _____
_____
_____
_____

> MY GOAL FOR THE 8-WEEK CHALLENGE: _____
_____
_____
_____

> MY LIFETIME GOAL: _____
_____
_____
_____

> I WANT TO FEEL: _____
_____
_____
_____
_____

Signature:_____

8-Week Workout Chart

Start>date_____ Finish>date_____

	Monday	Tuesday	Wednesday	Thursday	Friday	Saturday	Sunday
WEEK 1	DAY 1 PRIMARY WORKOUT ○	DAY 2 DAY OFF ○	DAY 3 DAY OFF ○	DAY 4 SECONDARY WORKOUT ○	DAY 5 DAY OFF ○	DAY 6 DAY OFF ○	DAY 7 DAY OFF ○
WEEK 2	DAY 8 PRIMARY WORKOUT ○	DAY 9 DAY OFF ○	DAY 10 DAY OFF ○	DAY 11 SECONDARY WORKOUT ○	DAY 12 DAY OFF ○	DAY 13 DAY OFF ○	DAY 14 DAY OFF ○
WEEK 3	DAY 15 PRIMARY WORKOUT ○	DAY 16 DAY OFF ○	DAY 17 DAY OFF ○	DAY 18 SECONDARY WORKOUT ○	DAY 19 DAY OFF ○	DAY 20 DAY OFF ○	DAY 21 DAY OFF ○
WEEK 4	DAY 22 PRIMARY WORKOUT ○	DAY 23 DAY OFF ○	DAY 24 DAY OFF ○	DAY 25 SECONDARY WORKOUT ○	DAY 26 DAY OFF ○	DAY 27 DAY OFF ○	DAY 28 DAY OFF ○
WEEK 5	DAY 29 PRIMARY WORKOUT ○	DAY 30 DAY OFF ○	DAY 31 DAY OFF ○	DAY 32 SECONDARY WORKOUT ○	DAY 33 DAY OFF ○	DAY 34 DAY OFF ○	DAY 35 DAY OFF ○
WEEK 6	DAY 36 PRIMARY WORKOUT ○	DAY 37 DAY OFF ○	DAY 38 DAY OFF ○	DAY 39 SECONDARY WORKOUT ○	DAY 40 DAY OFF ○	DAY 41 DAY OFF ○	DAY 42 DAY OFF ○
WEEK 7	DAY 43 PRIMARY WORKOUT ○	DAY 44 DAY OFF ○	DAY 45 DAY OFF ○	DAY 46 SECONDARY WORKOUT ○	DAY 47 DAY OFF ○	DAY 48 DAY OFF ○	DAY 49 DAY OFF ○
WEEK 8	DAY 50 PRIMARY WORKOUT ○	DAY 51 DAY OFF ○	DAY 52 DAY OFF ○	DAY 53 SECONDARY WORKOUT ○	DAY 54 DAY OFF ○	DAY 55 DAY OFF ○	DAY 56 SUCCESS! ●

*Please photocopy and place on your refrigerator. As you complete your workouts, cross off the days so you can see your success!

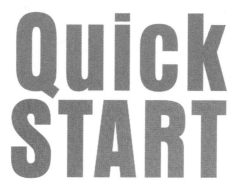

Quick START

The 12-Second Sequence™

This phase is designed to get you going fast. The workouts require absolutely *no* gym and can be done in your home. For the Quick Start phase, you'll need a set of dumbbells, a mat, and a Swiss ball. My favorites are made by a company called GoFit™. They're high-quality, affordable, and easy to find. If you have a gym membership, then of course you can do all the Quick Start workouts there. There's nothing wrong with that. But either way, there's no excuse not to get started!

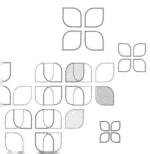

>>> A journey of a thousand miles must begin with a single step. —LAO-TZU

Jorge's Meditation > PREPARATION: Before you begin your 12-Second Sequence™ workouts, I want you to do a visualization exercise of what your life will be like when you make yourself a priority by focusing on your fitness and weight-loss goals. Do the following with me for just a few minutes: Close your eyes and take a few deep, relaxing breaths—in through your nose and out through your mouth. Imagine you have just woken up and it is the morning of your first workout. You stretch out your arms and legs and smile as you remember what day it is. What excites you about the prospect of changing your body? How will you feel after you've done something amazing and wonderful for your body? Will you stroll around outside? Hang out with your loved ones? Treat yourself with a warm bubble bath or a nice massage for making the commitment to improve your health and wellness? There are no limits to what you can do from here. You have the energy and zest for the life that you have been waiting for. Your muscles and bones feel healthy and your heart is brimming with love for yourself, the important people in your life, and, of course, for this new beginning.

DAY 1

DATE: _____

EATING PLANNER

This plan will ensure leaner muscle and a higher metabolism.

Breakfast>time_____

Description

○	PROTEIN* (3–5oz/40g)	
○	CARBS (½ cup or 1 slice of bread)	
○	FRUIT (1 cup)	
○	FAT (1 teaspoon)	

Snack>time_____

Description

○	WHEY PROTEIN SHAKE (1 scoop)	

Jorge recommends Jorge's Packs™ protein drinks. **>** See other recommended snacks at the back of the journal.

Lunch>time_____

Description

○	PROTEIN* (3–5oz/40g)	
○	CARBS (½ cup or 1 slice of bread)	
○	VEGGIES** (2 cups)	
○	FAT (1 teaspoon)	

Snack>time_____

Description

○	WHEY PROTEIN SHAKE (1 scoop)	

Dinner>time_____

Description

○	PROTEIN* (3–5oz/40g)	
○	VEGGIES** (2–4 cups)	
○	FAT (1 teaspoon)	

Snack>time_____

Description

○	WHEY PROTEIN SHAKE (1 scoop)	

*If you weigh under 150 pounds, eat 3 ounces of protein at every meal; if you weigh over 150 pounds, eat 5 ounces of protein.

**Veggies = nonstarchy vegetables.

Water (eight 8-oz cups) ○ ○ ○ ○ ○ ○ ○ ○

Multivitamin ○

WORKOUT LOG | WEEK_____ OF 8 |

Primary Workout

DATE_____ DAY_____ OF 56   Start>time_____ Finish>time_____

TOTAL TIME_____

Select weights so that by the end of the fourth rep of each exercise you feel an intensity level of 8.

CIRCUIT 1

Muscle Group	Exercise	Weight Used	Intensity Level
LEGS			
BACK			
CHEST			
ABS			

At this point you should be about 6 minutes into your workout.

CIRCUIT 2

Muscle Group	Exercise	Weight Used	Intensity Level
LEGS			
BACK			
CHEST			
ABS			

At this point you should be about 14 minutes into your workout, including 2 minutes of transition time.

CIRCUIT 3

Muscle Group	Exercise	Weight Used	Intensity Level
LEGS			
BACK			
CHEST			
ABS			

At this point in your workout you should be at 20 minutes. Congratulations! YOU DID IT!

BONUS CARDIO   26-MINUTE MORNING POWER WALK ○

After my workout I feel_____

(e.g., confident, strong)

< REFLECTIONS >

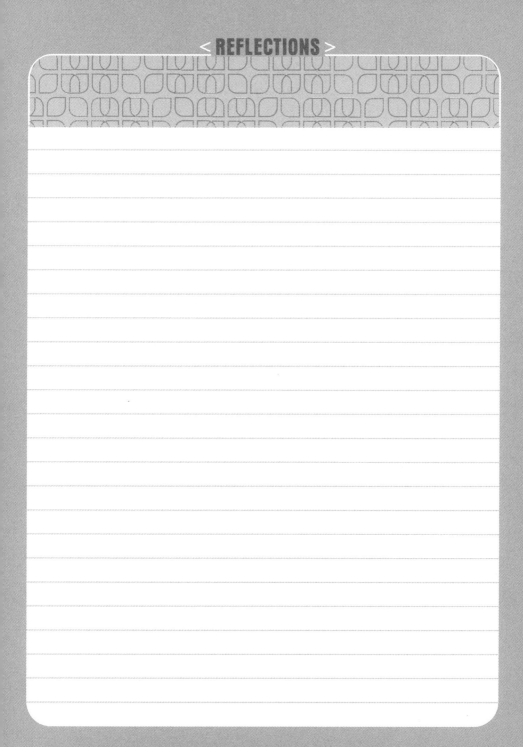

> > > Begin with the end in mind. —STEPHEN COVEY

Day Off! > NO WORKOUT TODAY

REFLECTIONS

_____

_____

_____

_____

_____

Jorge's Meditation > JOURNALING: This journal is going to be your touchstone as you journey through the 8-Week Challenge. Think of your journal as your own private, safe refuge, a place where you are free to express your innermost thoughts and feelings. Don't worry about grammar or writing in slang. Don't worry about always using the same color pen. All you need to do is let your feelings flow onto the pages. If you sit down and don't think you have anything to write about, that's fine—just write that. You might surprise yourself with where your writing goes from there. Think about your day. Look at your calendar if you need to remind yourself what you did. Do you feel good about your day? Did something happen, or not happen, that has been bothering you? What did you accomplish today? How have your eating habits been? Did you connect with other people? How did they make you feel? By simply recounting your day, you can discover so much about your feelings and what events trigger certain emotions. Each entry that you write in your journal brings you one step closer to truly knowing the real, strong, successful you!

BONUS CARDIO 26-MINUTE MORNING POWER WALK ○

DATE: _____

EATING PLANNER

This plan will ensure leaner muscle and a higher metabolism.

Breakfast>time_____   Description

○	PROTEIN* (3–5oz/40g)	
○	CARBS (½ cup or 1 slice of bread)	
○	FRUIT (1 cup)	
○	FAT (1 teaspoon)	

Snack>time_____   Description

○	WHEY PROTEIN SHAKE (1 scoop)	

Jorge recommends Jorge's Packs™ protein drinks. **>** See other recommended snacks at the back of the journal.

Lunch>time_____   Description

○	PROTEIN* (3–5oz/40g)	
○	CARBS (½ cup or 1 slice of bread)	
○	VEGGIES** (2 cups)	
○	FAT (1 teaspoon)	

Snack>time_____   Description

○	WHEY PROTEIN SHAKE (1 scoop)	

Dinner>time_____   Description

○	PROTEIN* (3–5oz/40g)	
○	VEGGIES** (2–4 cups)	
○	FAT (1 teaspoon)	

Snack>time_____   Description

○	WHEY PROTEIN SHAKE (1 scoop)	

*If you weigh under 150 pounds, eat 3 ounces of protein at every meal; if you weigh over 150 pounds, eat 5 ounces of protein.

**Veggies = nonstarchy vegetables.

Water (eight 8-oz cups) ○ ○ ○ ○ ○ ○ ○ ○

Multivitamin ○

> > > Obstacles are those frightful things you see when you take your eyes off your goal. —HENRY FORD

Day Off! > NO WORKOUT TODAY

REFLECTIONS

_____

_____

_____

_____

Jorge's Meditation > STRENGTH TRAINING: Regardless of your age, you can improve your health and your level of physical fitness. In fact, extensive research has shown that age-related decline in strength and motor skills can be significantly reduced through weight training, and it is never too late to rebuild muscle strength. Strength training can actually slow down or even reverse the aging process. You see, strength is a crucial component of any individual's quality of life and without it even the most basic tasks become difficult or impossible without assistance. Muscle atrophy is one of the most significant factors in one's loss of functioning, and to be specific, the lack of forceful contraction plays a major role—if you don't use it, you lose it. To combat muscle atrophy at any age you have to lift weights; aerobic exercise doesn't help. The beneficial effects of strength training are improved walking speed, ability to easily rise from a chair and climb stairs, ability to carry out simple household tasks, and decreased frequency of falls. It doesn't matter how old you are, the 12-Second Sequence™ will work for you.

BONUS CARDIO 26-MINUTE MORNING POWER WALK ○

DATE: _____

EATING PLANNER

This plan will ensure leaner muscle and a higher metabolism.

Breakfast>time _____

Description

○	PROTEIN* (3–5oz/40g)	
○	CARBS (½ cup or 1 slice of bread)	
○	FRUIT (1 cup)	
○	FAT (1 teaspoon)	

Snack>time _____

Description

○	WHEY PROTEIN SHAKE (1 scoop)

Jorge recommends Jorge's Packs™ protein drinks. **>** See other recommended snacks at the back of the journal.

Lunch>time _____

Description

○	PROTEIN* (3–5oz/40g)	
○	CARBS (½ cup or 1 slice of bread)	
○	VEGGIES** (2 cups)	
○	FAT (1 teaspoon)	

Snack>time _____

Description

○	WHEY PROTEIN SHAKE (1 scoop)

Dinner>time _____

Description

○	PROTEIN* (3–5oz/40g)	
○	VEGGIES** (2–4 cups)	
○	FAT (1 teaspoon)	

Snack>time _____

Description

○	WHEY PROTEIN SHAKE (1 scoop)

*If you weigh under 150 pounds, eat 3 ounces of protein at every meal; if you weigh over 150 pounds, eat 5 ounces of protein.

**Veggies = nonstarchy vegetables.

Water (eight 8-oz cups) ○ ○ ○ ○ ○ ○ ○ ○

Multivitamin ○

> > > **When health is absent, wisdom cannot reveal itself, art cannot become manifest, strength cannot be exerted, wealth is useless, and reason is powerless.** —HEROPHILUS

Jorge's Meditation > STRONG BONES: You know that doing your 12-Second Sequence™ workouts will help you shed pounds and have a younger-looking body, but did you know that building muscle also makes you *feel* younger? By strength training, you are building muscle and burning fat all day long. With your metabolism revved up, you will notice an increase in energy that allows you to feel strong and stay motivated. Another benefit of strength training is that it builds and fortifies your bones. As bones age, they lose calcium and other minerals, which make them more porous and susceptible to breaking. Getting enough calcium is important, but strength training can also do amazing things for your bone health. Because strength training is a "weight-bearing" exercise, you will actually be enhancing the density and durability of your bones. Your joints will also feel the benefit, since strength training will make your muscles, ligaments, and tendons stronger. On top of all those benefits, as you see and feel yourself getting stronger, your self-confidence will be on the rise as well!

DATE:

EATING PLANNER

This plan will ensure leaner muscle and a higher metabolism.

Breakfast>time_____   Description

○	PROTEIN* (3–5oz/40g)	
○	CARBS (½ cup or 1 slice of bread)	
○	FRUIT (1 cup)	
○	FAT (1 teaspoon)	

Snack>time_____   Description

| ○ | WHEY PROTEIN SHAKE (1 scoop) | |

Jorge recommends Jorge's Packs™ protein drinks. **>** See other recommended snacks at the back of the journal.

Lunch>time_____   Description

○	PROTEIN* (3–5oz/40g)	
○	CARBS (½ cup or 1 slice of bread)	
○	VEGGIES** (2 cups)	
○	FAT (1 teaspoon)	

Snack>time_____   Description

| ○ | WHEY PROTEIN SHAKE (1 scoop) | |

Dinner>time_____   Description

○	PROTEIN* (3–5oz/40g)	
○	VEGGIES** (2–4 cups)	
○	FAT (1 teaspoon)	

Snack>time_____   Description

| ○ | WHEY PROTEIN SHAKE (1 scoop) | |

*If you weigh under 150 pounds, eat 3 ounces of protein at every meal; if you weigh over 150 pounds, eat 5 ounces of protein.

**Veggies = nonstarchy vegetables.

Water (eight 8-oz cups) ○ ○ ○ ○ ○ ○ ○ ○

Multivitamin ○

WORKOUT LOG | WEEK_____OF 8

Secondary Workout

DATE_____ DAY____ OF 56

Start>time_____ Finish>time_____

TOTAL TIME_____

Select weights so that by the end of the fourth rep of each exercise you feel an intensity level of 8.

CIRCUIT 1

Muscle Group	Exercise	Weight Used	Intensity Level
SHOULDERS			
BICEPS			
TRICEPS			
ABS			

At this point you should be about 6 minutes into your workout.

CIRCUIT 2

Muscle Group	Exercise	Weight Used	Intensity Level
SHOULDERS			
BICEPS			
TRICEPS			
ABS			

At this point you should be about 14 minutes into your workout, including 2 minutes of transition time.

CIRCUIT 3

Muscle Group	Exercise	Weight Used	Intensity Level
SHOULDERS			
BICEPS			
TRICEPS			
ABS			

At this point in your workout you should be at 20 minutes. Congratulations! YOU DID IT!

BONUS CARDIO 26-MINUTE MORNING POWER WALK ○

After my workout I feel_____

(e.g., confident, strong)

< REFLECTIONS >

>>> Time is your most precious commodity. Don't waste it. —JORGE CRUISE

Day Off! > NO WORKOUT TODAY

REFLECTIONS _____
_____
_____
_____
_____

Jorge's Meditation > MAKING TIME: Today I want you to think about the importance of time in your life. If there's something that everyone wants more of it's time—time with our families, friends, or even just a little more time for ourselves. Now, I want you to let go of the idea that achieving your best body ever is going to take you a lot of time. I want you to imagine making the absolute most of each minute, each second of the time you devote to your fitness. See yourself waving good-bye to those hours and hours of time you have been wasting at the gym and envision yourself spending just 20 minutes twice a week on your workouts. Imagine the amazing results you're going to see in front of you in the mirror; think of all the other things you'll be able to focus on in your life with all the free time you'll have.

BONUS CARDIO 26-MINUTE MORNING POWER WALK ○

DAY 5

DATE: _____

EATING PLANNER
This plan will ensure leaner muscle and a higher metabolism.

Breakfast>time_____   Description

○	PROTEIN* (3–5oz/40g)	
○	CARBS (½ cup or 1 slice of bread)	
○	FRUIT (1 cup)	
○	FAT (1 teaspoon)	

Snack>time_____   Description

○	WHEY PROTEIN SHAKE (1 scoop)	

Jorge recommends Jorge's Packs™ protein drinks. **>** See other recommended snacks at the back of the journal.

Lunch>time_____   Description

○	PROTEIN* (3–5oz/40g)	
○	CARBS (½ cup or 1 slice of bread)	
○	VEGGIES** (2 cups)	
○	FAT (1 teaspoon)	

Snack>time_____   Description

○	WHEY PROTEIN SHAKE (1 scoop)	

Dinner>time_____   Description

○	PROTEIN* (3–5oz/40g)	
○	VEGGIES** (2–4 cups)	
○	FAT (1 teaspoon)	

Snack>time_____   Description

○	WHEY PROTEIN SHAKE (1 scoop)	

*If you weigh under 150 pounds, eat 3 ounces of protein at every meal; if you weigh over 150 pounds, eat 5 ounces of protein.

**Veggies = nonstarchy vegetables.

Water (eight 8-oz cups) ○ ○ ○ ○ ○ ○ ○ ○

Multivitamin ○

> > > **The first step towards getting some-where is to decide that you are not going to stay where you are.** —JOHN PIERPONT MORGAN

Day Off! > **NO WORKOUT TODAY**

REFLECTIONS _____

_____

_____

_____

Jorge's Meditation > **EATING EVERY THREE HOURS:** Today I want you to visualize yourself committing to eating every three hours. Close your eyes and take a few deep, relaxing breaths—in through your nose and out through your mouth. Now I want you to start by seeing yourself never skipping breakfast again. Imagine yourself eating the most important meal of the day within an hour of waking, and feel yourself energized through the midmorning when normally you would feel drained of energy. After breakfast, I want you to visualize your protein shake three hours later, and then your lunch three hours after that. Envision yourself taking the steps to ensure this simple structure is implemented into your life. See yourself reaching the point where eating every three hours is a natural habit for you, like brushing your teeth.

BONUS CARDIO 26-MINUTE MORNING POWER WALK ○

DATE: _____

EATING PLANNER

This plan will ensure leaner muscle and a higher metabolism.

Breakfast>time_____

Description

○	PROTEIN* (3–5oz/40g)	
○	CARBS (½ cup or 1 slice of bread)	
○	FRUIT (1 cup)	
○	FAT (1 teaspoon)	

Snack>time_____

Description

○	WHEY PROTEIN SHAKE (1 scoop)	

Jorge recommends Jorge's Packs™ protein drinks. **>** See other recommended snacks at the back of the journal.

Lunch>time_____

Description

○	PROTEIN* (3–5oz/40g)	
○	CARBS (½ cup or 1 slice of bread)	
○	VEGGIES** (2 cups)	
○	FAT (1 teaspoon)	

Snack>time_____

Description

○	WHEY PROTEIN SHAKE (1 scoop)	

Dinner>time_____

Description

○	PROTEIN* (3–5oz/40g)	
○	VEGGIES** (2–4 cups)	
○	FAT (1 teaspoon)	

Snack>time_____

Description

○	WHEY PROTEIN SHAKE (1 scoop)	

*If you weigh under 150 pounds, eat 3 ounces of protein at every meal; if you weigh over 150 pounds, eat 5 ounces of protein.

**Veggies = nonstarchy vegetables.

Water (eight 8-oz cups) ○ ○ ○ ○ ○ ○ ○ ○

Multivitamin ○

> > > We've got two lives. The one we're given and the one we make. —KOBE YAMADA

Day Off! > NO WORKOUT TODAY

REFLECTIONS _____

_____

_____

_____

_____

Jorge's Meditation > SHAPELY, NOT BULKY: Many women are hesitant about strength training at first because they fear they will bulk up and look even bigger. But, ladies, I promise you, this won't happen, and, in fact, quite the opposite is true. You will burn calories during your 12-Second Sequence™ moves, and, yes, you will gain muscle. Remember, muscle speeds up your metabolism and burns fat. If you were to lose weight without doing strength-training exercises, you'd likely lose muscle along with fat and, with less muscle, slow down your metabolism. Also, keep in mind that while muscle is heavier than fat, it is also more compact, meaning it takes up less space, and thus so will you. As you develop muscle you will instantly notice that your clothes are not as snug. Female bodybuilders with he-man-like proportions lift extremely heavy weights to see big gains in muscle size and, in some cases, take steroids to add more bulk. Trust me! Your muscles will look firm, sexy, and shapely, not bulky.

BONUS CARDIO 26-MINUTE MORNING POWER WALK ○

DAY 7

DATE: _____

EATING PLANNER
This plan will ensure leaner muscle and a higher metabolism.

Breakfast>time_____

Description

○	PROTEIN* (3–5oz/40g)	
○	CARBS (½ cup or 1 slice of bread)	
○	FRUIT (1 cup)	
○	FAT (1 teaspoon)	

Snack>time_____

Description

○	WHEY PROTEIN SHAKE (1 scoop)	

Jorge recommends Jorge's Packs™ protein drinks. **>** See other recommended snacks at the back of the journal.

Lunch>time_____

Description

○	PROTEIN* (3–5oz/40g)	
○	CARBS (½ cup or 1 slice of bread)	
○	VEGGIES** (2 cups)	
○	FAT (1 teaspoon)	

Snack>time_____

Description

○	WHEY PROTEIN SHAKE (1 scoop)	

Dinner>time_____

Description

○	PROTEIN* (3–5oz/40g)	
○	VEGGIES** (2–4 cups)	
○	FAT (1 teaspoon)	

Snack>time_____

Description

○	WHEY PROTEIN SHAKE (1 scoop)	

*If you weigh under 150 pounds, eat 3 ounces of protein at every meal; if you weigh over 150 pounds, eat 5 ounces of protein.

**Veggies = nonstarchy vegetables.

Water (eight 8-oz cups) ○ ○ ○ ○ ○ ○ ○ ○

Multivitamin ○

> > > **If you wait for the perfect moment when all is safe and assured, it may never arrive. Mountains will not be climbed, races won, or lasting happiness achieved.** —MAURICE CHEVALIER

Jorge's Meditation > GETTING CREATIVE WITH RECIPES: Close your eyes and take a few deep, relaxing breaths—in through your nose and out through your mouth. Imagine you awoke this morning, performed your 20-minute workout, or did your morning walk, and now you're heading to the kitchen to prepare yourself a wholesome breakfast. Will you make the Steak and Eggs with Potato Hash (see recipe in *The 12-Second Sequence*™)? Will you enjoy a cup of green tea? Three hours later, it's time for your protein shake. What about lunch? Will you enjoy the Curried Chicken Salad in Lettuce Cups you prepared last night? Or will you have a salad and a lean turkey sandwich on whole grain bread from the deli downstairs? Three hours later it's time for another shake. Three hours later, you've got a dinner date. Decide which veggies will fill your plate, and think about how much the pureed cauliflower with a little butter and salt and pepper will taste just like your favorite mashed potatoes. Think of how great you'll feel when you skip the starchy carbs. What else will you have? Remember, food is fuel, so give your body what it needs.

DATE: _____

EATING PLANNER

This plan will ensure leaner muscle and a higher metabolism.

Breakfast>time_____   Description

○	PROTEIN* (3–5oz/40g)	
○	CARBS (½ cup or 1 slice of bread)	
○	FRUIT (1 cup)	
○	FAT (1 teaspoon)	

Snack>time_____   Description

○	WHEY PROTEIN SHAKE (1 scoop)	

Jorge recommends Jorge's Packs™ protein drinks. **>** See other recommended snacks at the back of the journal.

Lunch>time_____   Description

○	PROTEIN* (3–5oz/40g)	
○	CARBS (½ cup or 1 slice of bread)	
○	VEGGIES** (2 cups)	
○	FAT (1 teaspoon)	

Snack>time_____   Description

○	WHEY PROTEIN SHAKE (1 scoop)	

Dinner>time_____   Description

○	PROTEIN* (3–5oz/40g)	
○	VEGGIES** (2–4 cups)	
○	FAT (1 teaspoon)	

Snack>time_____   Description

○	WHEY PROTEIN SHAKE (1 scoop)	

*If you weigh under 150 pounds, eat 3 ounces of protein at every meal; if you weigh over 150 pounds, eat 5 ounces of protein.

**Veggies = nonstarchy vegetables.

Water (eight 8-oz cups) ○ ○ ○ ○ ○ ○ ○ ○

Multivitamin ○

WORKOUT LOG WEEK_____ OF 8

Primary Workout

DATE_____ DAY_____ OF 56

Start>time_____ Finish>time_____

TOTAL TIME_____

Select weights so that by the end of the fourth rep of each exercise you feel an intensity level of 8.

	Muscle Group	Exercise	Weight Used	Intensity Level
CIRCUIT 1	LEGS			
	BACK			
	CHEST			
	ABS			

At this point you should be about 6 minutes into your workout.

	Muscle Group	Exercise	Weight Used	Intensity Level
CIRCUIT 2	LEGS			
	BACK			
	CHEST			
	ABS			

At this point you should be about 14 minutes into your workout, including 2 minutes of transition time.

	Muscle Group	Exercise	Weight Used	Intensity Level
CIRCUIT 3	LEGS			
	BACK			
	CHEST			
	ABS			

At this point in your workout you should be at 20 minutes. Congratulations! YOU DID IT!

BONUS CARDIO 26-MINUTE MORNING POWER WALK ○

After my workout I feel_____

(e.g., confident, strong)

< REFLECTIONS >

> > > Energy and persistence conquer all things. —BENJAMIN FRANKLIN

Day Off! > NO WORKOUT TODAY

REFLECTIONS _____

_____

_____

_____

Jorge's Meditation > REV UP YOUR METABOLISM!: Many people have been misled into thinking that they can easily lose unwanted weight by starving themselves. That may be true, but when you lose weight this way you lose as much lean muscle tissue as you do fat! You see, your muscle tissue is your body's metabolic furnace, and every pound of muscle burns roughly 50 calories a day. So every pound of muscle that you lose by dieting means that your metabolism will slow by 50 calories a day. As your metabolism slows down, you'll have to eat less and less food to compensate, which will eventually become extremely difficult. As soon as you start eating normally again, your body will regain the weight you lost, but this time, it will nearly all go into your fat cells and your metabolism will stay just as sluggish. This is why many people who lose weight this way end up gaining back more than they originally lost. So how can you get your muscle tissue back and rev up your body's metabolic furnace? With my 12-Second Sequence™ strength-training program! Keep up the great work—it *will* pay off.

BONUS CARDIO   26-MINUTE MORNING POWER WALK ○

DATE:

EATING PLANNER
This plan will ensure leaner muscle and a higher metabolism.

Breakfast>time_____

Description

○ PROTEIN* (3–5oz/40g)	
○ CARBS (½ cup or 1 slice of bread)	
○ FRUIT (1 cup)	
○ FAT (1 teaspoon)	

Snack>time_____

Description

○ WHEY PROTEIN SHAKE (1 scoop)	

Jorge recommends Jorge's Packs™ protein drinks. > See other recommended snacks at the back of the journal.

Lunch>time_____

Description

○ PROTEIN* (3–5oz/40g)	
○ CARBS (½ cup or 1 slice of bread)	
○ VEGGIES** (2 cups)	
○ FAT (1 teaspoon)	

Snack>time_____

Description

○ WHEY PROTEIN SHAKE (1 scoop)	

Dinner>time_____

Description

○ PROTEIN* (3–5oz/40g)	
○ VEGGIES** (2–4 cups)	
○ FAT (1 teaspoon)	

Snack>time_____

Description

○ WHEY PROTEIN SHAKE (1 scoop)	

*If you weigh under 150 pounds, eat 3 ounces of protein at every meal; if you weigh over 150 pounds, eat 5 ounces of protein.

**Veggies = nonstarchy vegetables.

Water (eight 8-oz cups) ○ ○ ○ ○ ○ ○ ○ ○

Multivitamin ○

>>> Believe in yourself! Have faith in your abilities!

—NORMAN VINCENT PEALE

Day Off! > NO WORKOUT TODAY

REFLECTIONS

_____

_____

_____

_____

Jorge's Meditation > **BREATHING:** Breathing is key to increasing your energy and focus. Without enough oxygen, you become lethargic, tired, and depressed. However, when you increase your oxygen levels, you not only increase your energy level, but also dramatically improve your mood. Plain and simple, you just feel better! The secret behind effective breathing is learning how to _belly breathe._ Belly breathing is actually the primary foundation for yoga—people in India have been doing it for hundreds of years. You will love how it makes you feel. The key to belly breathing is to use your diaphragm, the dome-shaped muscle located under your lungs. When you breathe in, notice that your belly wants to expand. Let this happen, but don't force it. Then retract your belly as you exhale and move the used oxygen out of your lungs. Do your belly-breathing exercises all day long, especially when you feel tired and lethargic.

BONUS CARDIO 26-MINUTE MORNING POWER WALK ○

DATE:

EATING PLANNER

This plan will ensure leaner muscle and a higher metabolism.

Breakfast>time_____   Description

○	PROTEIN* (3–5oz/40g)	
○	CARBS (½ cup or 1 slice of bread)	
○	FRUIT (1 cup)	
○	FAT (1 teaspoon)	

Snack>time_____   Description

○	WHEY PROTEIN SHAKE (1 scoop)	

Jorge recommends Jorge's Packs™ protein drinks. **>** See other recommended snacks at the back of the journal.

Lunch>time_____   Description

○	PROTEIN* (3–5oz/40g)	
○	CARBS (½ cup or 1 slice of bread)	
○	VEGGIES** (2 cups)	
○	FAT (1 teaspoon)	

Snack>time_____   Description

○	WHEY PROTEIN SHAKE (1 scoop)	

Dinner>time_____   Description

○	PROTEIN* (3–5oz/40g)	
○	VEGGIES** (2–4 cups)	
○	FAT (1 teaspoon)	

Snack>time_____   Description

○	WHEY PROTEIN SHAKE (1 scoop)	

*If you weigh under 150 pounds, eat 3 ounces of protein at every meal; if you weigh over 150 pounds, eat 5 ounces of protein.

**Veggies = nonstarchy vegetables.

Water (eight 8-oz cups) ○ ○ ○ ○ ○ ○ ○ ○

Multivitamin ○

> > > **Go confidently in the direction of your dreams! Live the life you've imagined.**

—HENRY DAVID THOREAU

Jorge's Meditation > USE YOUR DISSATISFACTION: Have you ever been so angry, sad, or disappointed at something you had been doing that you finally said, "Enough, I will never do this again!"? Well, that's what you must do right now about living an unhealthy life. Get dissatisfied and then use it as one of the most valuable motivational tools there is. Think about how being unfit has cost you in your career, an intimate relationship, and your family relationships. How many activities have you missed out on because you physically couldn't partake in them or because you felt too ashamed or embarrassed about being out of shape to participate? Be honest with yourself. Explore each and every aspect of your life in which inactivity and overeating has held you back. Pick up your pen and let your dissatisfaction tumble out onto the pages of this journal. Once done, you'll have the genesis of your success right in front of you. These are the reasons why it is crucial that you change your life for good. Whenever you start to question whether or not you really need to work out or walk today, go directly to this page in your journal and read it. Make the dissatisfaction work for you.

DATE:

EATING PLANNER

This plan will ensure leaner muscle and a higher metabolism.

Breakfast>time_____   Description

○	PROTEIN* (3–5oz/40g)	
○	CARBS (½ cup or 1 slice of bread)	
○	FRUIT (1 cup)	
○	FAT (1 teaspoon)	

Snack>time_____   Description

○	WHEY PROTEIN SHAKE (1 scoop)	

Jorge recommends Jorge's Packs™ protein drinks. **>** See other recommended snacks at the back of the journal.

Lunch>time_____   Description

○	PROTEIN* (3–5oz/40g)	
○	CARBS (½ cup or 1 slice of bread)	
○	VEGGIES** (2 cups)	
○	FAT (1 teaspoon)	

Snack>time_____   Description

○	WHEY PROTEIN SHAKE (1 scoop)	

Dinner>time_____   Description

○	PROTEIN* (3–5oz/40g)	
○	VEGGIES** (2–4 cups)	
○	FAT (1 teaspoon)	

Snack>time_____   Description

○	WHEY PROTEIN SHAKE (1 scoop)	

*If you weigh under 150 pounds, eat 3 ounces of protein at every meal; if you weigh over 150 pounds, eat 5 ounces of protein.

**Veggies = nonstarchy vegetables.

Water (eight 8-oz cups) ○ ○ ○ ○ ○ ○ ○ ○

Multivitamin ○

12-Second Sequence™

WORKOUT LOG | WEEK_____OF 8

Secondary Workout

DATE_____ DAY_____ OF 56

Start>time_____ Finish>time_____

TOTAL TIME_____

Select weights so that by the end of the fourth rep of each exercise you feel an intensity level of 8.

	Muscle Group	Exercise	Weight Used	Intensity Level
CIRCUIT 1	SHOULDERS			
	BICEPS			
	TRICEPS			
	ABS			

At this point you should be about 6 minutes into your workout.

	Muscle Group	Exercise	Weight Used	Intensity Level
CIRCUIT 2	SHOULDERS			
	BICEPS			
	TRICEPS			
	ABS			

At this point you should be about 14 minutes into your workout, including 2 minutes of transition time.

	Muscle Group	Exercise	Weight Used	Intensity Level
CIRCUIT 3	SHOULDERS			
	BICEPS			
	TRICEPS			
	ABS			

At this point in your workout you should be at 20 minutes. Congratulations! YOU DID IT!

BONUS CARDIO 26-MINUTE MORNING POWER WALK ○

After my workout I feel_____

(e.g., confident, strong)

< REFLECTIONS >

> > > **What I am looking for is not out there; it is in me.** —HELEN KELLER

Day Off! > NO WORKOUT TODAY

REFLECTIONS

_____

_____

_____

_____

Jorge's Meditation > **PLANNING:** Every Sunday night I sit down with my calendar and organize my week. I fill in the meetings, appearances, and professional business I need to attend to, and also what personal priorities I need to make time for, like working out, spending time with friends, and, most importantly, quality time with my wife and kids. Setting weekly and daily goals is a very important factor in leading a healthy and happy life. When you don't prioritize, you go around in circles and don't get much of anything done. When you are planning your week, make sure to block off the time you need for your 12-Second Sequence™ workouts. Think about the healthy meals you will be eating each day and make a grocery list so you will have everything you need. Also, make sure to plan for time with your loved ones. Whether it's a Thursday-night date or walk around the neighborhood with your spouse or a half-hour phone conversation with your best friend, schedule it! The more prepared and organized you are for a healthy week, the better your chances are of succeeding.

BONUS CARDIO 26-MINUTE MORNING POWER WALK ○

DATE:

EATING PLANNER

This plan will ensure leaner muscle and a higher metabolism.

Breakfast>time_____   Description

○	PROTEIN* (3–5oz/40g)	
○	CARBS (½ cup or 1 slice of bread)	
○	FRUIT (1 cup)	
○	FAT (1 teaspoon)	

Snack>time_____   Description

○	WHEY PROTEIN SHAKE (1 scoop)	

Jorge recommends Jorge's Packs™ protein drinks. **>** See other recommended snacks at the back of the journal.

Lunch>time_____   Description

○	PROTEIN* (3–5oz/40g)	
○	CARBS (½ cup or 1 slice of bread)	
○	VEGGIES** (2 cups)	
○	FAT (1 teaspoon)	

Snack>time_____   Description

○	WHEY PROTEIN SHAKE (1 scoop)	

Dinner>time_____   Description

○	PROTEIN* (3–5oz/40g)	
○	VEGGIES** (2–4 cups)	
○	FAT (1 teaspoon)	

Snack>time_____   Description

○	WHEY PROTEIN SHAKE (1 scoop)	

*If you weigh under 150 pounds, eat 3 ounces of protein at every meal; if you weigh over 150 pounds, eat 5 ounces of protein.

**Veggies = nonstarchy vegetables.

Water (eight 8-oz cups) ○ ○ ○ ○ ○ ○ ○ ○

Multivitamin ○

> > > They can because they think they can. —VIRGIL

REFLECTIONS _____
_____
_____
_____

Jorge's Meditation > MAKING GREAT CHOICES AT NIGHT: While
you sleep, your body repairs and builds your lean muscle tissue into visibly long,
lean, shapely muscles. If you eat late at night, your body will have to spend its
energy digesting the food in your tummy and not recuperating your muscles.
And since your metabolism slows at night, the calories you eat late most likely
will not all be used up, therefore turning right into fat. (The one exception to
this, of course, is the protein shake I recommend for everyone at night. This protein will help your body repair itself and enhance lean muscle development.) So
how can you overcome these urges to eat at night? The most important thing is
to make sure you are eating enough during the course of the day. Remember,
skipping meals will slow down your metabolism and make you susceptible to
late-night binges. One of the most common reasons that people eat a lot at night
is not because they are hungry, but because they are bored, tired, lonely, or
depressed. Ask yourself if you are really hungry before you even step into the
kitchen. Call your friend and tell her what you are planning on eating.
Remember, feed your hungry heart first; the rest will fall into place.

BONUS CARDIO 26-MINUTE MORNING POWER WALK ○

DATE:

EATING PLANNER

This plan will ensure leaner muscle and a higher metabolism.

Breakfast>time_____   Description

○	PROTEIN* (3–5oz/40g)	
○	CARBS (½ cup or 1 slice of bread)	
○	FRUIT (1 cup)	
○	FAT (1 teaspoon)	

Snack>time_____   Description

○	WHEY PROTEIN SHAKE (1 scoop)	

Jorge recommends Jorge's Packs™ protein drinks. **>** See other recommended snacks at the back of the journal.

Lunch>time_____   Description

○	PROTEIN* (3–5oz/40g)	
○	CARBS (½ cup or 1 slice of bread)	
○	VEGGIES** (2 cups)	
○	FAT (1 teaspoon)	

Snack>time_____   Description

○	WHEY PROTEIN SHAKE (1 scoop)	

Dinner>time_____   Description

○	PROTEIN* (3–5oz/40g)	
○	VEGGIES** (2–4 cups)	
○	FAT (1 teaspoon)	

Snack>time_____   Description

○	WHEY PROTEIN SHAKE (1 scoop)	

*If you weigh under 150 pounds, eat 3 ounces of protein at every meal; if you weigh over 150 pounds, eat 5 ounces of protein.

**Veggies = nonstarchy vegetables.

Water (eight 8-oz cups) ○ ○ ○ ○ ○ ○ ○ ○

Multivitamin ○

> > > **Health is beauty, and the most perfect health is the most perfect beauty.** —WILLIAM SHENSTONE

Day Off! > NO WORKOUT TODAY

REFLECTIONS _____

_____

_____

_____

Jorge's Meditation > PROTEIN: Protein is the primary building block of all the tissues in your body—especially your lean muscle tissue. If you don't have enough protein in your diet, you are not providing your body with the materials it needs to build the lean muscle that's going to burn calories *all day long.* The key to getting 40 percent of your calories from protein (recommended in *The 12-Second Sequence*™) is to incorporate enough protein into each meal. Also, high-protein snacks can be a great way to satisfy hunger and give you a healthy serving of those powerful building blocks. Protein shakes are a quick and easy solution. Remember to review the source of your protein because some sources can be absorbed more efficiently by your body than others. See *The 12-Second Sequence*™ for a complete list of recommended protein sources.

BONUS CARDIO 26-MINUTE MORNING POWER WALK ○

DATE: _____

EATING PLANNER

This plan will ensure leaner muscle and a higher metabolism.

Breakfast>time_____

Description

○	PROTEIN* (3–5oz/40g)	
○	CARBS (½ cup or 1 slice of bread)	
○	FRUIT (1 cup)	
○	FAT (1 teaspoon)	

Snack>time_____

Description

○	WHEY PROTEIN SHAKE (1 scoop)	

Jorge recommends Jorge's Packs™ protein drinks. **>** See other recommended snacks at the back of the journal.

Lunch>time_____

Description

○	PROTEIN* (3–5oz/40g)	
○	CARBS (½ cup or 1 slice of bread)	
○	VEGGIES** (2 cups)	
○	FAT (1 teaspoon)	

Snack>time_____

Description

○	WHEY PROTEIN SHAKE (1 scoop)	

Dinner>time_____

Description

○	PROTEIN* (3–5oz/40g)	
○	VEGGIES** (2–4 cups)	
○	FAT (1 teaspoon)	

Snack>time_____

Description

○	WHEY PROTEIN SHAKE (1 scoop)	

*If you weigh under 150 pounds, eat 3 ounces of protein at every meal; if you weigh over 150 pounds, eat 5 ounces of protein.

**Veggies = nonstarchy vegetables.

Water (eight 8-oz cups) ○ ○ ○ ○ ○ ○ ○ ○

Multivitamin ○

< REFLECTIONS >

Advanced

The 12-Second Sequence™

For the first two weeks of the Advanced phase, you'll incorporate many new moves that will still require your dumbbells, mat, and Swiss ball. You can also continue to work out in your own home if that's where you're most comfortable. But things will change when we start week 5. To progressively challenge your muscles best you will need to start using a "functional trainer" (FT) cable machine when you reach week 5.

You can either go to a gym to use one (Bally Total Fitness™ is a great gym choice and will have a functional trainer at all of their locations) or purchase one for your home. Precor® makes a great one; the S3.23 is the one I use in my home gym. You can find more information about GoFit™, Bally Total Fitness™, and Precor® at www.12second.com.

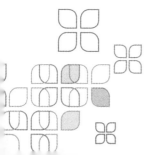

> > > **If we did all the things we are capable of doing, we would literally astound ourselves.**

—THOMAS EDISON

Jorge's Meditation > WATER: Not getting enough water can affect your body in so many ways—it can make you feel lazy, unmotivated, and tired; it can make your muscles tight, and can even slow the process of recovery after you work out. In fact, when your body is dehydrated, it can create a "false" hunger—meaning your body misinterprets thirst for hunger and you can end up overeating. To keep hydrated, I recommend drinking at least half of your body weight (in pounds) of water (in ounces) every day. For example, if you weigh 170 pounds, you should be drinking 85 ounces, or about ten-and-a-half 8-ounce glasses of water every day. I know that seems like a lot, but you can get creative with where you get your water. A great way is to try some water-filled foods. Some of the best food sources of water include apples, celery, cucumbers, 100 percent fruit juices, grapefruit, grapes, and watermelon. You can also try one of my favorite drinks, Propel® Fit Water™ by the makers of Gatorade®. They have lots of great flavors and they only have 10 calories per 8-ounce serving. Treat your body right and go grab a glass of water, a bunch of grapes, or a Propel® Fit Water™ right now!

DATE: _____

EATING PLANNER

This plan will ensure leaner muscle and a higher metabolism.

Breakfast>time_____   Description

○	PROTEIN* (3–5oz/40g)	
○	CARBS (½ cup or 1 slice of bread)	
○	FRUIT (1 cup)	
○	FAT (1 teaspoon)	

Snack>time_____   Description

○	WHEY PROTEIN SHAKE (1 scoop)	

Jorge recommends Jorge's Packs™ protein drinks. **>** See other recommended snacks at the back of the journal.

Lunch>time_____   Description

○	PROTEIN* (3–5oz/40g)	
○	CARBS (½ cup or 1 slice of bread)	
○	VEGGIES** (2 cups)	
○	FAT (1 teaspoon)	

Snack>time_____   Description

○	WHEY PROTEIN SHAKE (1 scoop)	

Dinner>time_____   Description

○	PROTEIN* (3–5oz/40g)	
○	VEGGIES** (2–4 cups)	
○	FAT (1 teaspoon)	

Snack>time_____   Description

○	WHEY PROTEIN SHAKE (1 scoop)	

*If you weigh under 150 pounds, eat 3 ounces of protein at every meal; if you weigh over 150 pounds, eat 5 ounces of protein.

**Veggies = nonstarchy vegetables.

Water (eight 8-oz cups) ○ ○ ○ ○ ○ ○ ○ ○

Multivitamin ○

WORKOUT LOG
WEEK_____ OF 8

Primary Workout

DATE_____ DAY_____ OF 56

Start>time_____ Finish>time_____

TOTAL TIME_____

Select weights so that by the end of the fourth rep of each exercise you feel an intensity level of 8.

	Muscle Group	Exercise	Weight Used	Intensity Level
CIRCUIT 1	LEGS			
	BACK			
	CHEST			
	ABS			

At this point you should be about 6 minutes into your workout.

	Muscle Group	Exercise	Weight Used	Intensity Level
CIRCUIT 2	LEGS			
	BACK			
	CHEST			
	ABS			

At this point you should be about 14 minutes into your workout, including 2 minutes of transition time.

	Muscle Group	Exercise	Weight Used	Intensity Level
CIRCUIT 3	LEGS			
	BACK			
	CHEST			
	ABS			

At this point in your workout you should be at 20 minutes. Congratulations! YOU DID IT!

BONUS CARDIO 26-MINUTE MORNING POWER WALK ○

After my workout I feel_____

(e.g., confident, strong)

< REFLECTIONS >

> > > **I believe that one of life's greatest risks is never daring to risk.**

—OPRAH WINFREY

Day Off! > **NO WORKOUT TODAY**

REFLECTIONS _____
_____
_____
_____
_____

Jorge's Meditation > THE NEW YOU: Now that you've embarked on the road to a healthier new you, I know that you will never turn back. Many of my clients are so excited about the knowledge they've discovered about living life to the fullest that they want to know even more. I encourage you to keep learning everything you can about your body, nutrition, exercise, science, vitamins— anything that will maintain and invigorate your ongoing success. There are many great resources out there that can provide you with wonderful information, inspiration, and guidance. From books and magazines to websites and seminars, I encourage you to build a resource library of your own. Look back at how much you've learned since you started my program and how far that knowledge has taken you. Knowledge is truly power, so keep on learning!

BONUS CARDIO 26-MINUTE MORNING POWER WALK ○

DATE:

EATING PLANNER

This plan will ensure leaner muscle and a higher metabolism.

Breakfast>time_____   Description

○	PROTEIN* (3–5oz/40g)	
○	CARBS (½ cup or 1 slice of bread)	
○	FRUIT (1 cup)	
○	FAT (1 teaspoon)	

Snack>time_____   Description

○	WHEY PROTEIN SHAKE (1 scoop)	

Jorge recommends Jorge's Packs™ protein drinks. > See other recommended snacks at the back of the journal.

Lunch>time_____   Description

○	PROTEIN* (3–5oz/40g)	
○	CARBS (½ cup or 1 slice of bread)	
○	VEGGIES** (2 cups)	
○	FAT (1 teaspoon)	

Snack>time_____   Description

○	WHEY PROTEIN SHAKE (1 scoop)	

Dinner>time_____   Description

○	PROTEIN* (3–5oz/40g)	
○	VEGGIES** (2–4 cups)	
○	FAT (1 teaspoon)	

Snack>time_____   Description

○	WHEY PROTEIN SHAKE (1 scoop)	

*If you weigh under 150 pounds, eat 3 ounces of protein at every meal; if you weigh over 150 pounds, eat 5 ounces of protein.

**Veggies = nonstarchy vegetables.

Water (eight 8-oz cups) ○ ○ ○ ○ ○ ○ ○ ○

Multivitamin ○

>>> Our aspirations are our possibilities.

—ROBERT BROWNING

Day Off! > NO WORKOUT TODAY

REFLECTIONS _____
_____
_____
_____
_____

Jorge's Meditation > LEAN MUSCLE TISSUE: Today I want you to think about how your beautiful lean muscle is transforming your body. Do the following with me for just a few minutes: Close your eyes and take a few deep, relaxing breaths—in through your nose and out through your mouth. I want you to imagine the long, lean, shapely muscle tissue as it sculpts your best body ever. Think about its amazing calorie-burning power—every pound of muscle you put on your body works overtime consuming an extra 50 calories a day, even when you're doing nothing at all. Imagine the compact, lean muscle tissue replacing unwanted fat on your body. See it changing the shape of your body. Envision your waist as it continues to shrink and feel the looseness in your jeans as you slip them on. It feels great!

BONUS CARDIO 26-MINUTE MORNING POWER WALK ○

DATE: _____

EATING PLANNER
This plan will ensure leaner muscle and a higher metabolism.

Breakfast>time_____   Description

○	PROTEIN* (3–5oz/40g)	
○	CARBS (½ cup or 1 slice of bread)	
○	FRUIT (1 cup)	
○	FAT (1 teaspoon)	

Snack>time_____   Description

○	WHEY PROTEIN SHAKE (1 scoop)	

Jorge recommends Jorge's Packs™ protein drinks. **>** See other recommended snacks at the back of the journal.

Lunch>time_____   Description

○	PROTEIN* (3–5oz/40g)	
○	CARBS (½ cup or 1 slice of bread)	
○	VEGGIES** (2 cups)	
○	FAT (1 teaspoon)	

Snack>time_____   Description

○	WHEY PROTEIN SHAKE (1 scoop)	

Dinner>time_____   Description

○	PROTEIN* (3–5oz/40g)	
○	VEGGIES** (2–4 cups)	
○	FAT (1 teaspoon)	

Snack>time_____   Description

○	WHEY PROTEIN SHAKE (1 scoop)	

*If you weigh under 150 pounds, eat 3 ounces of protein at every meal; if you weigh over 150 pounds, eat 5 ounces of protein.

**Veggies = nonstarchy vegetables.

Water (eight 8-oz cups) ○ ○ ○ ○ ○ ○ ○ ○

Multivitamin ○

> > > **Your body is your vehicle for life. As long as you are here, live in it. Love, honor, respect and cherish it, treat it well, and it will serve you in kind.** —SUZY PRUDDEN

Jorge's Meditation > A FRESH START WITH FOOD: Since beginning your 12-Second Sequence™ program, has the kitchen become your friend or foe? If you feel uncomfortable about cooking now that you're not eating the fattening foods that you're used to whipping up, or if you've never felt quite at home in a chef's hat, it's time to give it a fresh start. Just like an artist, you can't get to work in the kitchen without the right tools and know-how. Here are some culinary tips that will help you get cooking right: Buy a good set of knives. You can optimize your dicing and slicing time by using the right 8- to 10-inch chef's knife. Before you buy a knife, pick it up and see if it feels comfortable in your hand and is a balanced weight that you can handle. Also, it's a good idea to invest in a knife sharpener to keep your knives at their sharpest. Nothing stinks more than trying to cut a tomato or loaf of bread with a dull knife.

DATE: _____

EATING PLANNER

This plan will ensure leaner muscle and a higher metabolism.

Breakfast>time_____   Description

○	PROTEIN* (3–5oz/40g)	
○	CARBS (½ cup or 1 slice of bread)	
○	FRUIT (1 cup)	
○	FAT (1 teaspoon)	

Snack>time_____   Description

| ○ | WHEY PROTEIN SHAKE (1 scoop) | |

Jorge recommends Jorge's Packs™ protein drinks. > See other recommended snacks at the back of the journal.

Lunch>time_____   Description

○	PROTEIN* (3–5oz/40g)	
○	CARBS (½ cup or 1 slice of bread)	
○	VEGGIES** (2 cups)	
○	FAT (1 teaspoon)	

Snack>time_____   Description

| ○ | WHEY PROTEIN SHAKE (1 scoop) | |

Dinner>time_____   Description

○	PROTEIN* (3–5oz/40g)	
○	VEGGIES** (2–4 cups)	
○	FAT (1 teaspoon)	

Snack>time_____   Description

| ○ | WHEY PROTEIN SHAKE (1 scoop) | |

*If you weigh under 150 pounds, eat 3 ounces of protein at every meal; if you weigh over 150 pounds, eat 5 ounces of protein.

**Veggies = nonstarchy vegetables.

Water (eight 8-oz cups) ○ ○ ○ ○ ○ ○ ○ ○

Multivitamin ○

WORKOUT LOG

WEEK_____ OF 8

Secondary Workout

DATE_____ DAY_____ OF 56

Start>time_____ Finish>time_____

TOTAL TIME_____

Select weights so that by the end of the fourth rep of each exercise you feel an intensity level of 8.

CIRCUIT 1

Muscle Group	Exercise	Weight Used	Intensity Level
SHOULDERS			
BICEPS			
TRICEPS			
ABS			

At this point you should be about 6 minutes into your workout.

CIRCUIT 2

Muscle Group	Exercise	Weight Used	Intensity Level
SHOULDERS			
BICEPS			
TRICEPS			
ABS			

At this point you should be about 14 minutes into your workout, including 2 minutes of transition time.

CIRCUIT 3

Muscle Group	Exercise	Weight Used	Intensity Level
SHOULDERS			
BICEPS			
TRICEPS			
ABS			

At this point in your workout you should be at 20 minutes. Congratulations! YOU DID IT!

BONUS CARDIO 26-MINUTE MORNING POWER WALK ○

After my workout I feel_____

(e.g., confident, strong)

> > > Things may come to those who wait, but only the things left by those who hustle. —ABRAHAM LINCOLN

Day Off! > **NO WORKOUT TODAY**

REFLECTIONS _____

_____

_____

_____

Jorge's Meditation > **INTENSITY:** Now that you've discovered that you can get an amazing workout in just 20 minutes with the 12-Second Sequence™, I want you to imagine yourself taking it up a notch. Today I want you to do a visualization exercise where you see yourself raising the intensity level. Close your eyes and take a few deep, relaxing breaths—in through your nose and out through your mouth. Now imagine yourself counting through the last 10 seconds of your first exercise; feel the muscles in your legs as you finish the last rep of your lunges. Feel your legs begin to shake a little bit and the sweat form on the back of your knees. Now reach into your deepest source of strength and motivation and count slowly through the last 5 seconds. Focus on your lean muscle and feel it pushing you through the final part of the exercise. Feel your lean muscle changing your body. Take hold of this level of intensity and carry it with you through all your exercises. This intensity is what will create your best body ever.

BONUS CARDIO 26-MINUTE MORNING POWER WALK ○

DATE:

EATING PLANNER

This plan will ensure leaner muscle and a higher metabolism.

Breakfast>time_____   Description

○	**PROTEIN*** (3–5oz/40g)
○	**CARBS** (½ cup or 1 slice of bread)
○	**FRUIT** (1 cup)
○	**FAT** (1 teaspoon)

Snack>time_____   Description

○	**WHEY PROTEIN SHAKE** (1 scoop)

Jorge recommends Jorge's Packs™ protein drinks. **>** See other recommended snacks at the back of the journal.

Lunch>time_____   Description

○	**PROTEIN*** (3–5oz/40g)
○	**CARBS** (½ cup or 1 slice of bread)
○	**VEGGIES**** (2 cups)
○	**FAT** (1 teaspoon)

Snack>time_____   Description

○	**WHEY PROTEIN SHAKE** (1 scoop)

Dinner>time_____   Description

○	**PROTEIN*** (3–5oz/40g)
○	**VEGGIES**** (2–4 cups)
○	**FAT** (1 teaspoon)

Snack>time_____   Description

○	**WHEY PROTEIN SHAKE** (1 scoop)

*If you weigh under 150 pounds, eat 3 ounces of protein at every meal; if you weigh over 150 pounds, eat 5 ounces of protein.

**Veggies = nonstarchy vegetables.

Water (eight 8-oz cups) ○ ○ ○ ○ ○ ○ ○ ○

Multivitamin ○

> > > **Don't say, "If I could, I would." Say, "If I can, I will."** —JIM ROHN

20

Day Off! > NO WORKOUT TODAY

REFLECTIONS _____

_____

_____

_____

Jorge's Meditation > BE ADVENTUROUS!: How many fitness programs have you tried—and failed—because they required you to eat the same foods every day, give up the foods you love, and do the same exercise the same way every day? Well, you might have figured out that deprivation and lack of new experiences is downright boring and not the key to lasting weight loss. What does work? Living life with a sense of purpose and adventure: experimenting with new foods, trying new activities, meeting new people, and looking at yourself and the world in a whole new light. By making simple, small changes, you can add adventure to your life and be excited to wake up every morning. To maintain your sense of adventure, try seeking out one new experience every day. It could be as simple as trying a vegetable you've never had before or saying hello to your neighbor for the first time. Check out a new magazine, website, or TV program. The more you read, watch, and learn about different ideas, people, and cultures, the more your world will expand.

BONUS CARDIO 26-MINUTE MORNING POWER WALK ○

DATE: _____

EATING PLANNER

This plan will ensure leaner muscle and a higher metabolism.

Breakfast>time_____   Description

○	PROTEIN* (3–5oz/40g)	
○	CARBS (½ cup or 1 slice of bread)	
○	FRUIT (1 cup)	
○	FAT (1 teaspoon)	

Snack>time_____   Description

| ○ | WHEY PROTEIN SHAKE (1 scoop) | |

Jorge recommends Jorge's Packs™ protein drinks. **>** See other recommended snacks at the back of the journal.

Lunch>time_____   Description

○	PROTEIN* (3–5oz/40g)	
○	CARBS (½ cup or 1 slice of bread)	
○	VEGGIES** (2 cups)	
○	FAT (1 teaspoon)	

Snack>time_____   Description

| ○ | WHEY PROTEIN SHAKE (1 scoop) | |

Dinner>time_____   Description

○	PROTEIN* (3–5oz/40g)	
○	VEGGIES** (2–4 cups)	
○	FAT (1 teaspoon)	

Snack>time_____   Description

| ○ | WHEY PROTEIN SHAKE (1 scoop) | |

*If you weigh under 150 pounds, eat 3 ounces of protein at every meal; if you weigh over 150 pounds, eat 5 ounces of protein.

**Veggies = nonstarchy vegetables.

Water (eight 8-oz cups) ○ ○ ○ ○ ○ ○ ○ ○

Multivitamin ○

>>> It's time to start living the life you've imagined.

—HENRY JAMES

Day Off! > NO WORKOUT TODAY

REFLECTIONS

_____

_____

_____

_____

Jorge's Meditation > FEATHERED BREATHING: Breathing properly can help calm your nerves, stabilize your emotions, and keep you alert. Even more importantly, breathing properly while you exercise can keep your body energized through an entire workout. You see, when you exercise, your muscles need oxygen to keep going. With the 12-Second Sequence™, it's important to remember to use the feathered breathing technique. This means you take a deep breath when you start any exercise and then follow with short bursts through your exhale. Whenever you get stressed throughout your day, try breathing through your nose. When you breathe in and out through your mouth, you risk not getting enough oxygen to the brain, and your body naturally responds by speeding up your breathing. Take a few deep breaths through your nose to regulate the flow of carbon dioxide and oxygen and keep your mind and body charged—you'll immediately feel cool, calm, and collected.

BONUS CARDIO 26-MINUTE MORNING POWER WALK ○

DATE:

EATING PLANNER

This plan will ensure leaner muscle and a higher metabolism.

Breakfast>time_____   Description

○	**PROTEIN*** (3–5oz/40g)	
○	**CARBS** (½ cup or 1 slice of bread)	
○	**FRUIT** (1 cup)	
○	**FAT** (1 teaspoon)	

Snack>time_____   Description

○	**WHEY PROTEIN SHAKE** (1 scoop)

Jorge recommends Jorge's Packs™ protein drinks. **>** See other recommended snacks at the back of the journal.

Lunch>time_____   Description

○	**PROTEIN*** (3–5oz/40g)	
○	**CARBS** (½ cup or 1 slice of bread)	
○	**VEGGIES**** (2 cups)	
○	**FAT** (1 teaspoon)	

Snack>time_____   Description

○	**WHEY PROTEIN SHAKE** (1 scoop)

Dinner>time_____   Description

○	**PROTEIN*** (3–5oz/40g)	
○	**VEGGIES**** (2–4 cups)	
○	**FAT** (1 teaspoon)	

Snack>time_____   Description

○	**WHEY PROTEIN SHAKE** (1 scoop)

*If you weigh under 150 pounds, eat 3 ounces of protein at every meal; if you weigh over 150 pounds, eat 5 ounces of protein.

**Veggies = nonstarchy vegetables.

Water (eight 8-oz cups) ○ ○ ○ ○ ○ ○ ○ ○

Multivitamin ○

> > > **Failure is not failure to meet your goal. Real failure is failure to reach as high as you possibly can.** —ROBERT SCHULLER

Jorge's Meditation > ENSURED SUCCESS: If you've had any trouble getting your workout in, try doing it first thing in the morning. You'll increase your metabolism for the rest of the day and release endorphins into your body, which means you'll be in a better mood when dealing with coworkers or your kids, and you'll reduce your blood pressure. But the most crucial reason might be the fact that the morning time is when you are the least likely to talk yourself out of it. The morning is simply the time of the day that is the easiest to control. Not many people have excuses like unexpected meetings, last-minute dates, or can't-miss opportunities early in the morning. When you put exercising off for later in the day, there's a good chance it will never get done. Distractions can— and will—come up, and I guarantee if given the choice of helping your child with his homework, snuggling on the couch with your spouse, surfing the Net for a little longer, *or* exercising, your dumbbells will get dusty. So make the morning the time you commit to yourself. I know you will have a better day because of it and enjoy every minute with your loved ones all the more.

DATE: _____

EATING PLANNER

This plan will ensure leaner muscle and a higher metabolism.

Breakfast>time _____   Description

○	**PROTEIN*** (3–5oz/40g)	
○	**CARBS** (½ cup or 1 slice of bread)	
○	**FRUIT** (1 cup)	
○	**FAT** (1 teaspoon)	

Snack>time _____   Description

○	**WHEY PROTEIN SHAKE** (1 scoop)	

Jorge recommends Jorge's Packs™ protein drinks. **>** See other recommended snacks at the back of the journal.

Lunch>time _____   Description

○	**PROTEIN*** (3–5oz/40g)	
○	**CARBS** (½ cup or 1 slice of bread)	
○	**VEGGIES**** (2 cups)	
○	**FAT** (1 teaspoon)	

Snack>time _____   Description

○	**WHEY PROTEIN SHAKE** (1 scoop)	

Dinner>time _____   Description

○	**PROTEIN*** (3–5oz/40g)	
○	**VEGGIES**** (2–4 cups)	
○	**FAT** (1 teaspoon)	

Snack>time _____   Description

○	**WHEY PROTEIN SHAKE** (1 scoop)	

*If you weigh under 150 pounds, eat 3 ounces of protein at every meal; if you weigh over 150 pounds, eat 5 ounces of protein.

**Veggies = nonstarchy vegetables.

Water (eight 8-oz cups) ○ ○ ○ ○ ○ ○ ○ ○

Multivitamin ○

WORKOUT LOG | WEEK_____ OF 8

Primary Workout

DATE_____ DAY____ OF 56

Start>time_____ Finish>time_____

TOTAL TIME_____

Select weights so that by the end of the fourth rep of each exercise you feel an intensity level of 8.

	Muscle Group	Exercise	Weight Used	Intensity Level
CIRCUIT 1	LEGS			
	BACK			
	CHEST			
	ABS			

At this point you should be about 6 minutes into your workout.

CIRCUIT 2	LEGS			
	BACK			
	CHEST			
	ABS			

At this point you should be about 14 minutes into your workout, including 2 minutes of transition time.

CIRCUIT 3	LEGS			
	BACK			
	CHEST			
	ABS			

At this point in your workout you should be at 20 minutes. Congratulations! YOU DID IT!

BONUS CARDIO 26-MINUTE MORNING POWER WALK ○

After my workout I feel_____

(e.g., confident, strong)

< REFLECTIONS >

>>> Whether you think you can or you think you can't, you're right. —HENRY FORD

Day Off! > NO WORKOUT TODAY

REFLECTIONS _____

_____

_____

_____

_____

Jorge's Meditation > NEVER LOOK BACK: Today I want you to think about moving forward with your new 12-Second Sequence™ lifestyle. I want you to visualize the changes you've made and everything you've implemented into your life, from new foods to a new way of thinking about exercise. I want you to think about the healthful choices you are now making and the commitment you've made to living a longer, better life. Imagine this transformation as you would a baby who learns to walk after crawling for a long time. You now have the tools to walk and experience your life from a new perspective—and you will never return to crawling. See yourself living this incredible new life and continuing forward with more confidence, a slimmer waist, more energy, and a whole new outlook on life.

BONUS CARDIO 26-MINUTE MORNING POWER WALK ○

DATE:

EATING PLANNER

This plan will ensure leaner muscle and a higher metabolism.

Breakfast>time_____   Description

○	PROTEIN* (3–5oz/40g)	
○	CARBS (½ cup or 1 slice of bread)	
○	FRUIT (1 cup)	
○	FAT (1 teaspoon)	

Snack>time_____   Description

○	WHEY PROTEIN SHAKE (1 scoop)	

Jorge recommends Jorge's Packs™ protein drinks. **>** See other recommended snacks at the back of the journal.

Lunch>time_____   Description

○	PROTEIN* (3–5oz/40g)	
○	CARBS (½ cup or 1 slice of bread)	
○	VEGGIES** (2 cups)	
○	FAT (1 teaspoon)	

Snack>time_____   Description

○	WHEY PROTEIN SHAKE (1 scoop)	

Dinner>time_____   Description

○	PROTEIN* (3–5oz/40g)	
○	VEGGIES** (2–4 cups)	
○	FAT (1 teaspoon)	

Snack>time_____   Description

○	WHEY PROTEIN SHAKE (1 scoop)	

*If you weigh under 150 pounds, eat 3 ounces of protein at every meal; if you weigh over 150 pounds, eat 5 ounces of protein.

**Veggies = nonstarchy vegetables.

Water (eight 8-oz cups) ○ ○ ○ ○ ○ ○ ○ ○

Multivitamin ○

>>> Every day is a new life. Seize it. Live it.
—DAVID GUY POWERS

Day Off! > NO WORKOUT TODAY

REFLECTIONS _____
_____
_____
_____

Jorge's Meditation > BUDDY SYSTEM/PEOPLE SOLUTION: Making sure you have the support of people around you is the number-one secret of my most successful clients. If you already have a solid group of friends and family around you, make sure they are aware of the commitment you've made to yourself—this way you can rely on them to offer encouraging words during challenging times. If you aren't getting the support you need in your life, try joining our online club at 12second.com. This is an online community that is available twenty-four hours a day. These online friends can become your e-mail and phone buddies and can help keep you going strong throughout the 8-Week Challenge. Remember, you can also post your before picture there and track your measurements and weight progress throughout the eight weeks and beyond. Whatever you do, make sure you have many safety nets set up to help you stay motivated through any rough spots. We all need a little bit of encouragement and support sometimes!

BONUS CARDIO 26-MINUTE MORNING POWER WALK ○

DATE:

EATING PLANNER

This plan will ensure leaner muscle and a higher metabolism.

Breakfast>time_____   Description

○	PROTEIN* (3–5oz/40g)	
○	CARBS (½ cup or 1 slice of bread)	
○	FRUIT (1 cup)	
○	FAT (1 teaspoon)	

Snack>time_____   Description

○	WHEY PROTEIN SHAKE (1 scoop)	

Jorge recommends Jorge's Packs™ protein drinks. **>** See other recommended snacks at the back of the journal.

Lunch>time_____   Description

○	PROTEIN* (3–5oz/40g)	
○	CARBS (½ cup or 1 slice of bread)	
○	VEGGIES** (2 cups)	
○	FAT (1 teaspoon)	

Snack>time_____   Description

○	WHEY PROTEIN SHAKE (1 scoop)	

Dinner>time_____   Description

○	PROTEIN* (3–5oz/40g)	
○	VEGGIES** (2–4 cups)	
○	FAT (1 teaspoon)	

Snack>time_____   Description

○	WHEY PROTEIN SHAKE (1 scoop)	

*If you weigh under 150 pounds, eat 3 ounces of protein at every meal; if you weigh over 150 pounds, eat 5 ounces of protein.

**Veggies = nonstarchy vegetables.

Water (eight 8-oz cups) ○ ○ ○ ○ ○ ○ ○ ○

Multivitamin ○

> > > **The person who makes a success of living is the one who sees his goal steadily and aims for it unswervingly.** —CECIL B. DeMILLE

Jorge's Meditation > MIDWAY PICTURE: Once you've lost weight and focused on your fitness, you are not free to overindulge, forget about drinking your protein shakes, or revert to a life without exercise. One of the best ways to keep your motivation up is to take a midway picture and compare it to your before shot. Under each picture, write down the traits or qualities that you feel or see that are associated with each time in your life. How did you feel then and how do you feel now? Don't allow yourself to be overly critical halfway through the 8-Week Challenge. Many people become overly sensitive about each part of their body as they begin to lose weight because they begin to focus too intently on small imperfections that they didn't even notice before. You are just more aware of your body, and that is a good thing, but you have to work that awareness in a positive light. Focus on how it feels physically, as well as emotionally, to be at this weight. You need to get your inner dialogue in touch with the way you look on the outside. Remember, achieving a healthy lifestyle is a process, not a destination, and you need to continuously work at feeling great.

DATE: _____

EATING PLANNER

This plan will ensure leaner muscle and a higher metabolism.

Breakfast>time_____   Description

○	PROTEIN* (3–5oz/40g)	
○	CARBS (½ cup or 1 slice of bread)	
○	FRUIT (1 cup)	
○	FAT (1 teaspoon)	

Snack>time_____   Description

○	WHEY PROTEIN SHAKE (1 scoop)	

Jorge recommends Jorge's Packs™ protein drinks. > See other recommended snacks at the back of the journal.

Lunch>time_____   Description

○	PROTEIN* (3–5oz/40g)	
○	CARBS (½ cup or 1 slice of bread)	
○	VEGGIES** (2 cups)	
○	FAT (1 teaspoon)	

Snack>time_____   Description

○	WHEY PROTEIN SHAKE (1 scoop)	

Dinner>time_____   Description

○	PROTEIN* (3–5oz/40g)	
○	VEGGIES** (2–4 cups)	
○	FAT (1 teaspoon)	

Snack>time_____   Description

○	WHEY PROTEIN SHAKE (1 scoop)	

*If you weigh under 150 pounds, eat 3 ounces of protein at every meal; if you weigh over 150 pounds, eat 5 ounces of protein.

**Veggies = nonstarchy vegetables.

Water (eight 8-oz cups) ○ ○ ○ ○ ○ ○ ○ ○

Multivitamin ○

WORKOUT LOG | WEEK_____OF 8

Secondary Workout

DATE_____ DAY_____ OF 56

Start>time_____ Finish>time_____

TOTAL TIME_____

Select weights so that by the end of the fourth rep of each exercise you feel an intensity level of 8.

	Muscle Group	Exercise	Weight Used	Intensity Level
CIRCUIT 1	SHOULDERS			
	BICEPS			
	TRICEPS			
	ABS			

At this point you should be about 6 minutes into your workout.

	Muscle Group	Exercise	Weight Used	Intensity Level
CIRCUIT 2	SHOULDERS			
	BICEPS			
	TRICEPS			
	ABS			

At this point you should be about 14 minutes into your workout, including 2 minutes of transition time.

	Muscle Group	Exercise	Weight Used	Intensity Level
CIRCUIT 3	SHOULDERS			
	BICEPS			
	TRICEPS			
	ABS			

At this point in your workout you should be at 20 minutes. Congratulations! YOU DID IT!

BONUS CARDIO 26-MINUTE MORNING POWER WALK ○

After my workout I feel_____

(e.g., confident, strong)

< REFLECTIONS >

> > > **Optimisim is the faith that leads to achievement. Nothing can be done without hope and confidence.** —HELEN KELLER

Day Off! > NO WORKOUT TODAY

REFLECTIONS _____

_____

_____

_____

Jorge's Meditation > **REWARD YOURSELF:** You should have your 8-Week Challenge end date marked on your calendar. In addition to this date, add mini goals along the way that you can reward yourself for. These goals can include completing your two weekly strength-training sessions, walking every day, losing 5 pounds, or even just writing in this journal. Remember, your reward can be anything, and it should be something you love that supports your new healthy lifestyle. Some great rewards are any type of pampering, like a massage, facial, manicure, or pedicure; a day at the beach; a healthy new cookbook; aromatherapy candles or bubble bath; a new outfit or pair of shoes; a new CD; or anything else that you can think of and afford. Remember, rewards were meant to be reaped, so keep up the good work.

BONUS CARDIO 26-MINUTE MORNING POWER WALK ○

DATE: _____

EATING PLANNER

This plan will ensure leaner muscle and a higher metabolism.

Breakfast>time_____   Description

○	PROTEIN* (3–5oz/40g)	
○	CARBS (½ cup or 1 slice of bread)	
○	FRUIT (1 cup)	
○	FAT (1 teaspoon)	

Snack>time_____   Description

○	WHEY PROTEIN SHAKE (1 scoop)	

Jorge recommends Jorge's Packs™ protein drinks. **>** See other recommended snacks at the back of the journal.

Lunch>time_____   Description

○	PROTEIN* (3–5oz/40g)	
○	CARBS (½ cup or 1 slice of bread)	
○	VEGGIES** (2 cups)	
○	FAT (1 teaspoon)	

Snack>time_____   Description

○	WHEY PROTEIN SHAKE (1 scoop)	

Dinner>time_____   Description

○	PROTEIN* (3–5oz/40g)	
○	VEGGIES** (2–4 cups)	
○	FAT (1 teaspoon)	

Snack>time_____   Description

○	WHEY PROTEIN SHAKE (1 scoop)	

*If you weigh under 150 pounds, eat 3 ounces of protein at every meal; if you weigh over 150 pounds, eat 5 ounces of protein.

**Veggies = nonstarchy vegetables.

Water (eight 8-oz cups) ○ ○ ○ ○ ○ ○ ○ ○

Multivitamin ○

> > > **The difference between the impossible and the possible lies in a person's determination.**

—TOMMY LASORDA

Day Off! > NO WORKOUT TODAY

REFLECTIONS _____

_____

_____

_____

Jorge's Meditation > MAKE THE MOST OF YOUR JOURNAL: You should be writing in this journal whenever you feel stressed, angry, sad, tense, depressed, guilty, or alone, and whenever you feel the urge to skip your workout or sabotage your commitment to the eating plan. To get even more from your journaling experience, you can expand your notebook to include special sections where you record different aspects of your 8-Week Challenge. You might add a section for special issues that you are exploring, like creative positive rewards for yourself or overcoming negative thinking. You can write and expand your ideas about each special subject whenever you have a new experience, perception, or insight. This can help you discover patterns and solutions to your special issues one word at a time.

BONUS CARDIO 26-MINUTE MORNING POWER WALK ○

DATE:

EATING PLANNER

This plan will ensure leaner muscle and a higher metabolism.

Breakfast>time_____   Description

○	PROTEIN* (3–5oz/40g)	
○	CARBS (½ cup or 1 slice of bread)	
○	FRUIT (1 cup)	
○	FAT (1 teaspoon)	

Snack>time_____   Description

○	WHEY PROTEIN SHAKE (1 scoop)	

Jorge recommends Jorge's Packs™ protein drinks. **>** See other recommended snacks at the back of the journal.

Lunch>time_____   Description

○	PROTEIN* (3–5oz/40g)	
○	CARBS (½ cup or 1 slice of bread)	
○	VEGGIES** (2 cups)	
○	FAT (1 teaspoon)	

Snack>time_____   Description

○	WHEY PROTEIN SHAKE (1 scoop)	

Dinner>time_____   Description

○	PROTEIN* (3–5oz/40g)	
○	VEGGIES** (2–4 cups)	
○	FAT (1 teaspoon)	

Snack>time_____   Description

○	WHEY PROTEIN SHAKE (1 scoop)	

*If you weigh under 150 pounds, eat 3 ounces of protein at every meal; if you weigh over 150 pounds, eat 5 ounces of protein.

**Veggies = nonstarchy vegetables.

Water (eight 8-oz cups) ○ ○ ○ ○ ○ ○ ○ ○

Multivitamin ○

> > > **Take care of your body. It's the only place you have to live.** —JIM ROHN

Day Off! > NO WORKOUT TODAY

REFLECTIONS

_____

_____

_____

_____

Jorge's Meditation > GET ENOUGH SLEEP!: Being able to wake up rested and ready for your day is not the only reason why adequate sleep is crucial to achieving your fitness goals. Research has found that getting too few zzzs may also be the reason why so many of us overeat. The logic behind this theory is that when you don't get enough sleep, it makes it harder for your body to push fat and sugar into the cells that burn them for energy. And consistently not getting enough sleep can actually raise the stress hormone cortisol, which can bring on a prediabetic state. At the same time, inadequate sleep lowers your levels of leptin, the hormone that decreases your appetite. What does all this mean in layman's terms? Your body will signal to you that it needs more energy to function. And what will this signal feel like? Hunger and intense cravings for sweets and starches. And what happens if you give in to these cravings? Your insulin levels will soar and then quickly crash. This amounts to mood swings, stress, sadness, impatience, aggravation, and, ultimately, another food binge. Why do this to your body?

BONUS CARDIO 26-MINUTE MORNING POWER WALK ○

DATE: _____

EATING PLANNER

This plan will ensure leaner muscle and a higher metabolism.

Breakfast>time_____   Description

○	**PROTEIN*** (3–5oz/40g)	
○	**CARBS** (½ cup or 1 slice of bread)	
○	**FRUIT** (1 cup)	
○	**FAT** (1 teaspoon)	

Snack>time_____   Description

○	**WHEY PROTEIN SHAKE** (1 scoop)	

Jorge recommends Jorge's Packs™ protein drinks. **>** See other recommended snacks at the back of the journal.

Lunch>time_____   Description

○	**PROTEIN*** (3–5oz/40g)	
○	**CARBS** (½ cup or 1 slice of bread)	
○	**VEGGIES**** (2 cups)	
○	**FAT** (1 teaspoon)	

Snack>time_____   Description

○	**WHEY PROTEIN SHAKE** (1 scoop)	

Dinner>time_____   Description

○	**PROTEIN*** (3–5oz/40g)	
○	**VEGGIES**** (2–4 cups)	
○	**FAT** (1 teaspoon)	

Snack>time_____   Description

○	**WHEY PROTEIN SHAKE** (1 scoop)	

*If you weigh under 150 pounds, eat 3 ounces of protein at every meal; if you weigh over 150 pounds, eat 5 ounces of protein.

**Veggies = nonstarchy vegetables.

Water (eight 8-oz cups) ○ ○ ○ ○ ○ ○ ○ ○

Multivitamin ○

> > > **When you whole-heartedly adopt a "with all your heart" attitude and go out with the positive principle, you can do incredible things.** —NORMAN VINCENT PEALE

Jorge's Meditation > A LOOK INTO THE FUTURE: Close your eyes and take a few deep, relaxing breaths—in through your nose and out through your mouth. Imagine you are getting ready for a very special date. Whoever your date is, he or she is very lucky to be with you as you hit the town for a romantic evening of dinner and dancing. How do you prepare for your date? Perhaps by taking a hot bubble bath with a glass of champagne? See yourself picking something beautiful out of your closet to wear and laying it out on your bed. As you pull the garment on, notice how the fabric touches against your smooth skin. Now it's time to do your hair and makeup. Notice how much firmer your face is and how much younger you look! You hear the doorbell ring and eager butterflies dance through your tummy as you stride confidently toward the door. When you open it, your date's eyes light up at how lovely you look. As you go out on the town, imagine how wonderful you feel. And best of all, how do you feel dancing the night away, so light on your feet? Last, but not least, when your date drops you off at your house, might there be a good-night kiss?

DATE: _____

EATING PLANNER

This plan will ensure leaner muscle and a higher metabolism.

Breakfast>time_____   Description

○	PROTEIN* (3–5oz/40g)	
○	CARBS (½ cup or 1 slice of bread)	
○	FRUIT (1 cup)	
○	FAT (1 teaspoon)	

Snack>time_____   Description

○	WHEY PROTEIN SHAKE (1 scoop)	

Jorge recommends Jorge's Packs™ protein drinks. **>** See other recommended snacks at the back of the journal.

Lunch>time_____   Description

○	PROTEIN* (3–5oz/40g)	
○	CARBS (½ cup or 1 slice of bread)	
○	VEGGIES** (2 cups)	
○	FAT (1 teaspoon)	

Snack>time_____   Description

○	WHEY PROTEIN SHAKE (1 scoop)	

Dinner>time_____   Description

○	PROTEIN* (3–5oz/40g)	
○	VEGGIES** (2–4 cups)	
○	FAT (1 teaspoon)	

Snack>time_____   Description

○	WHEY PROTEIN SHAKE (1 scoop)	

*If you weigh under 150 pounds, eat 3 ounces of protein at every meal; if you weigh over 150 pounds, eat 5 ounces of protein.

**Veggies = nonstarchy vegetables.

Water (eight 8-oz cups) ○ ○ ○ ○ ○ ○ ○ ○

Multivitamin ○

WORKOUT LOG
WEEK_____ OF 8

Primary Workout

DATE_____ DAY_____ OF 56

Start>time_____ Finish>time_____

TOTAL TIME_____

Select weights so that by the end of the fourth rep of each exercise you feel an intensity level of 8.

	Muscle Group	Exercise	Weight Used	Intensity Level
CIRCUIT 1	LEGS			
	BACK			
	CHEST			
	ABS			

At this point you should be about 6 minutes into your workout.

	Muscle Group	Exercise	Weight Used	Intensity Level
CIRCUIT 2	LEGS			
	BACK			
	CHEST			
	ABS			

At this point you should be about 14 minutes into your workout, including 2 minutes of transition time.

	Muscle Group	Exercise	Weight Used	Intensity Level
CIRCUIT 3	LEGS			
	BACK			
	CHEST			
	ABS			

At this point in your workout you should be at 20 minutes. Congratulations! YOU DID IT!

BONUS CARDIO 26-MINUTE MORNING POWER WALK ○

After my workout I feel_____

(e.g., confident, strong)

< REFLECTIONS >

> > > **You have to believe in yourself when no one else does—that makes you a winner right there.**

—VENUS WILLIAMS

Day Off! > NO WORKOUT TODAY

REFLECTIONS _____

_____

_____

_____

Jorge's Meditation > **KEEP A POSITIVE ATTITUDE:** With all the negative messages our society is bombarded with every day, it is so important to counter the negatives with powerful, positive statements. There are tons of positive affirmation books and calendars available at bookstores, but I think it is important, and kind of fun, to write your own. Make sure you recite your affirmations out loud several times a day. You can use them over and over or even pass them on to your buddies. When writing your own affirmations, remember to use the vocabulary of success. Don't use words like *should, hope,* or *try.* Instead use words like *will, must, can,* and *know.* Here are some examples of positive affirmations to get you started: "I accept myself just as I am." "I know that I have the power to choose a healthy lifestyle." "I can take the time to nourish my body and mind."

BONUS CARDIO 26-MINUTE MORNING POWER WALK ○

DATE:

EATING PLANNER
This plan will ensure leaner muscle and a higher metabolism.

Breakfast>time_____   Description

○	**PROTEIN*** (3–5oz/40g)	
○	**CARBS** (½ cup or 1 slice of bread)	
○	**FRUIT** (1 cup)	
○	**FAT** (1 teaspoon)	

Snack>time_____   Description

○	**WHEY PROTEIN SHAKE** (1 scoop)	

Jorge recommends Jorge's Packs™ protein drinks. **>** See other recommended snacks at the back of the journal.

Lunch>time_____   Description

○	**PROTEIN*** (3–5oz/40g)	
○	**CARBS** (½ cup or 1 slice of bread)	
○	**VEGGIES**** (2 cups)	
○	**FAT** (1 teaspoon)	

Snack>time_____   Description

○	**WHEY PROTEIN SHAKE** (1 scoop)	

Dinner>time_____   Description

○	**PROTEIN*** (3–5oz/40g)	
○	**VEGGIES**** (2–4 cups)	
○	**FAT** (1 teaspoon)	

Snack>time_____   Description

○	**WHEY PROTEIN SHAKE** (1 scoop)	

*If you weigh under 150 pounds, eat 3 ounces of protein at every meal; if you weigh over 150 pounds, eat 5 ounces of protein.

**Veggies = nonstarchy vegetables.

Water (eight 8-oz cups) ○ ○ ○ ○ ○ ○ ○ ○
Multivitamin ○

>>> Whatever you can do, or dream you can, begin it.

—GOETHE

Day Off! > NO WORKOUT TODAY

REFLECTIONS _____

_____

_____

_____

Jorge's Meditation > **EXPRESS YOURSELF:** There will always be people and situations that upset your equilibrium even when you've reached your goal weight. In many instances, your anger or frustration might be completely justified, but it's up to you to react in a positive, healthy manner—a manner that doesn't involve eating food. So what is the "right" way to be angry? Well, it's best to express your feelings in a calm and rational manner that yields constructive results. Many people don't verbalize their anger and they often turn to food to ease their emotional hurt. Instead, you must confront your anger and work through it with others. Start small and practice confronting family members about little things that anger you. Use "I" sentences and be specific in letting others know how their actions made you feel. For example, instead of saying "You never make me feel appreciated," try saying "I feel frustrated and hurt when you do not acknowledge me for picking up your dry cleaning." Avoid insults and sarcasm when you are explaining how you feel; if you're getting too emotional with someone, make a plan to talk at a later time when you're calmer.

BONUS CARDIO   26-MINUTE MORNING POWER WALK ○

DATE:

EATING PLANNER

This plan will ensure leaner muscle and a higher metabolism.

Breakfast>time_____   Description

○	**PROTEIN*** (3–5oz/40g)	
○	**CARBS** (½ cup or 1 slice of bread)	
○	**FRUIT** (1 cup)	
○	**FAT** (1 teaspoon)	

Snack>time_____   Description

○	**WHEY PROTEIN SHAKE** (1 scoop)	

Jorge recommends Jorge's Packs™ protein drinks. **>** See other recommended snacks at the back of the journal.

Lunch>time_____   Description

○	**PROTEIN*** (3–5oz/40g)	
○	**CARBS** (½ cup or 1 slice of bread)	
○	**VEGGIES**** (2 cups)	
○	**FAT** (1 teaspoon)	

Snack>time_____   Description

○	**WHEY PROTEIN SHAKE** (1 scoop)	

Dinner>time_____   Description

○	**PROTEIN*** (3–5oz/40g)	
○	**VEGGIES**** (2–4 cups)	
○	**FAT** (1 teaspoon)	

Snack>time_____   Description

○	**WHEY PROTEIN SHAKE** (1 scoop)	

*If you weigh under 150 pounds, eat 3 ounces of protein at every meal; if you weigh over 150 pounds, eat 5 ounces of protein.

**Veggies = nonstarchy vegetables.

Water (eight 8-oz cups) ○ ○ ○ ○ ○ ○ ○ ○

Multivitamin ○

> > > **Obstacles don't have to stop you. If you run into a wall, don't turn around and give up. Figure out how to climb it, go through it, or work around it.** —MICHAEL JORDAN

Jorge's Meditation > POSTURE: Posture is one of the most overlooked, yet most important, aspects of our appearance. Hunching over while you stand or sit not only makes you look heavier, but it also makes you feel heavier! Just by sitting up straight, you can look and feel like a happier, more vigorous and confident person, while also easing tension in your back and neck. Here are some daily reminder exercises that you can use to keep your posture in check: Hang a mirror by your desk where you can't see your reflection unless you are slumped forward in bad posture. Whenever you see yourself in the mirror, straighten up! Every time you stand up, picture your body parts as blocks that you stack to create your long, lean silhouette. Your spinal vertebrae should stack in a straight line, and your ears, shoulders, hips, knees, and ankles should all fall into alignment. Stick brightly colored tape at the level your eyes should be if you're sitting up straight. Whenever you notice the tape, make sure you're in line with it. Check your posture at your desk at work to make sure that you sit up straight. Standing and walking tall will not only make you look better, but also make you feel more attractive and sure of yourself.

DATE:

EATING PLANNER

This plan will ensure leaner muscle and a higher metabolism.

Breakfast>time_____   Description

○	PROTEIN* (3–5oz/40g)	
○	CARBS (½ cup or 1 slice of bread)	
○	FRUIT (1 cup)	
○	FAT (1 teaspoon)	

Snack>time_____   Description

○	WHEY PROTEIN SHAKE (1 scoop)	

Jorge recommends Jorge's Packs™ for your protein drinks. > See list of other recommended snacks at the back.

Lunch>time_____   Description

○	PROTEIN* (3–5oz/40g)	
○	CARBS (½ cup or 1 slice of bread)	
○	VEGGIES** (2 cups)	
○	FAT (1 teaspoon)	

Snack>time_____   Description

○	WHEY PROTEIN SHAKE (1 scoop)	

Dinner>time_____   Description

○	PROTEIN* (3–5oz/40g)	
○	VEGGIES** (2–4 cups)	
○	FAT (1 teaspoon)	

Snack>time_____   Description

○	WHEY PROTEIN SHAKE (1 scoop)	

*If you weigh under 150 pounds, eat 3 ounces of protein at every meal; if you weigh over 150 pounds, eat 5 ounces of protein.

**Veggies = nonstarchy vegetables.

Water (eight 8-oz cups) ○ ○ ○ ○ ○ ○ ○ ○

Multivitamin ○

WORKOUT LOG | WEEK_____ OF 8

Secondary Workout

DATE_____ DAY_____ OF 56

Start>time_____ Finish>time_____

TOTAL TIME_____

Select weights so that by the end of the fourth rep of each exercise you feel an intensity level of 8.

	Muscle Group	Exercise	Weight Used	Intensity Level
CIRCUIT 1	SHOULDERS			
	BICEPS			
	TRICEPS			
	ABS			

At this point you should be about 6 minutes into your workout.

	Muscle Group	Exercise	Weight Used	Intensity Level
CIRCUIT 2	SHOULDERS			
	BICEPS			
	TRICEPS			
	ABS			

At this point you should be about 14 minutes into your workout, including 2 minutes of transition time.

	Muscle Group	Exercise	Weight Used	Intensity Level
CIRCUIT 3	SHOULDERS			
	BICEPS			
	TRICEPS			
	ABS			

At this point in your workout you should be at 20 minutes. Congratulations! YOU DID IT!

BONUS CARDIO 26-MINUTE MORNING POWER WALK ○

After my workout I feel_____

(e.g., confident, strong)

< REFLECTIONS >

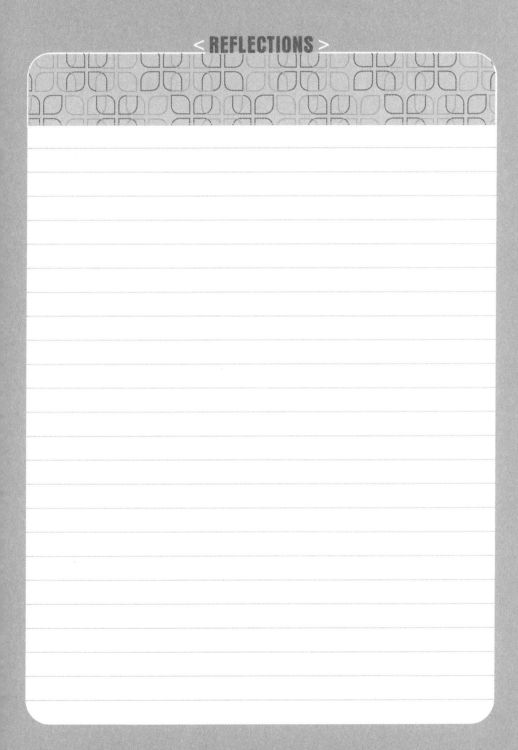

> > > **Life is short.
Live it well.** —JORGE CRUISE

Day Off! > **NO WORKOUT TODAY**

REFLECTIONS _____

_____

_____

_____

Jorge's Meditation > **BE CONFIDENT!:** Have you ever missed out on meeting a new person just because you were too shy to approach him or her? The first thing you need to do is stop telling yourself that you are a shy person. Do it now! Tell yourself that you are confident and attractive and that people enjoy spending time with you, and it will become your reality. You are who you think you are; it's as simple as that. Next, stock your mind with conversation starters to use when you meet someone for the first time. In most social situations, fear comes from being put on the spot and not being able to come up with something to say, or even worse, saying the wrong thing. If you have a couple of general questions in mind ahead of time, you will be ready. Try easy questions such as "How do you know the host of the party?" Questions like this will get you and a stranger talking face-to-face in a nonthreatening way. Giving a genuine compliment is another way to start a conversation. Try to relax and really listen to the intent behind the other person's words. Above all, don't forget the power of good eye contact and a warm, gracious smile.

BONUS CARDIO 26-MINUTE MORNING POWER WALK ○

DATE: _____

EATING PLANNER

This plan will ensure leaner muscle and a higher metabolism.

Breakfast>time_____   Description

○ PROTEIN* (3–5oz/40g)	
○ CARBS (½ cup or 1 slice of bread)	
○ FRUIT (1 cup)	
○ FAT (1 teaspoon)	

Snack>time_____   Description

○ WHEY PROTEIN SHAKE (1 scoop)	

Jorge recommends Jorge's Packs™ protein drinks. **>** See other recommended snacks at the back of the journal.

Lunch>time_____   Description

○ PROTEIN* (3–5oz/40g)	
○ CARBS (½ cup or 1 slice of bread)	
○ VEGGIES** (2 cups)	
○ FAT (1 teaspoon)	

Snack>time_____   Description

○ WHEY PROTEIN SHAKE (1 scoop)	

Dinner>time_____   Description

○ PROTEIN* (3–5oz/40g)	
○ VEGGIES** (2–4 cups)	
○ FAT (1 teaspoon)	

Snack>time_____   Description

○ WHEY PROTEIN SHAKE (1 scoop)	

*If you weigh under 150 pounds, eat 3 ounces of protein at every meal; if you weigh over 150 pounds, eat 5 ounces of protein.

**Veggies = nonstarchy vegetables.

Water (eight 8-oz cups) ○ ○ ○ ○ ○ ○ ○ ○
Multivitamin ○

> > > There is no such thing in anyone's life as an unimportant day.

—ALEXANDER WOOLLCOTT

Day Off! > **NO WORKOUT TODAY**

REFLECTIONS _____

_____

_____

_____

_____

Jorge's Meditation > **GRACIOUSNESS IS AN ART:** How did you react the last time someone gave you a compliment? If you said something along the lines of "Oh, come on . . . you're lying," "Oh, hush," or "I'm not what you think I am," then you are not fully respecting your body. Remember, you need to accept and respect your body unconditionally right now. Even if you feel that the person giving you the compliment is trying to flatter you, don't turn it into something bad about yourself. The best answer to a compliment is "Thank you." To reject a compliment is to reject the bearer of that compliment. Being gracious is an art and it makes the person who gives the compliment feel good. When you give a compliment, be sincere. A sincere compliment makes all of us feel appreciated, but flattery is telling people what they want to hear even when you know it isn't true. So avoid saying something that you don't really mean.

BONUS CARDIO 26-MINUTE MORNING POWER WALK ○

DATE:

EATING PLANNER

This plan will ensure leaner muscle and a higher metabolism.

Breakfast>time_____   Description

○	PROTEIN* (3–5oz/40g)	
○	CARBS (½ cup or 1 slice of bread)	
○	FRUIT (1 cup)	
○	FAT (1 teaspoon)	

Snack>time_____   Description

| ○ | WHEY PROTEIN SHAKE (1 scoop) | |

Jorge recommends Jorge's Packs™ protein drinks. **>** See other recommended snacks at the back of the journal.

Lunch>time_____   Description

○	PROTEIN* (3–5oz/40g)	
○	CARBS (½ cup or 1 slice of bread)	
○	VEGGIES** (2 cups)	
○	FAT (1 teaspoon)	

Snack>time_____   Description

| ○ | WHEY PROTEIN SHAKE (1 scoop) | |

Dinner>time_____   Description

○	PROTEIN* (3–5oz/40g)	
○	VEGGIES** (2–4 cups)	
○	FAT (1 teaspoon)	

Snack>time_____   Description

| ○ | WHEY PROTEIN SHAKE (1 scoop) | |

*If you weigh under 150 pounds, eat 3 ounces of protein at every meal; if you weigh over 150 pounds, eat 5 ounces of protein.

**Veggies = nonstarchy vegetables.

Water (eight 8-oz cups) ○ ○ ○ ○ ○ ○ ○ ○

Multivitamin ○

> > > Never, never, in nothing great or small, large or petty, never give in except to convictions of honor and good sense. —WINSTON CHURCHILL

Day Off! > NO WORKOUT TODAY

REFLECTIONS _____
_____
_____
_____

Jorge's Meditation > AVOID NEGATIVE ENERGY: There are times in all of our lives when strangers will offend us. People who snub and attack others are terribly insecure people who have very empty, hungry hearts. So how should you react to these unfortunate individuals? Well, there is a Chinese proverb that says it is better to ignore an insult than to respond to one. I think there is much wisdom in that. By failing to notice or give any sort of reaction to an insult, you're not allowing that person to triumph with their comment or action. This is not to say that you should be a rug and let everyone walk all over you. On the contrary, by making the decision not to let an insult affect you, you are showcasing your confidence and self-respect.

BONUS CARDIO 26-MINUTE MORNING POWER WALK ○

DATE: _____

EATING PLANNER

This plan will ensure leaner muscle and a higher metabolism.

Breakfast>time_____   Description

○	PROTEIN* (3–5oz/40g)	
○	CARBS (½ cup or 1 slice of bread)	
○	FRUIT (1 cup)	
○	FAT (1 teaspoon)	

Snack>time_____   Description

○	WHEY PROTEIN SHAKE (1 scoop)	

Jorge recommends Jorge's Packs™ protein drinks. **>** See other recommended snacks at the back of the journal.

Lunch>time_____   Description

○	PROTEIN* (3–5oz/40g)	
○	CARBS (½ cup or 1 slice of bread)	
○	VEGGIES** (2 cups)	
○	FAT (1 teaspoon)	

Snack>time_____   Description

○	WHEY PROTEIN SHAKE (1 scoop)	

Dinner>time_____   Description

○	PROTEIN* (3–5oz/40g)	
○	VEGGIES** (2–4 cups)	
○	FAT (1 teaspoon)	

Snack>time_____   Description

○	WHEY PROTEIN SHAKE (1 scoop)	

*If you weigh under 150 pounds, eat 3 ounces of protein at every meal; if you weigh over 150 pounds, eat 5 ounces of protein.

**Veggies = nonstarchy vegetables.

Water (eight 8-oz cups) ○ ○ ○ ○ ○ ○ ○ ○

Multivitamin ○

> > > **Energy is the essence of life. Every day you decide how you're going to use it by knowing what you want and what it takes to reach that goal, and by maintaining focus.**

—OPRAH WINFREY

Jorge's Meditation > YOUR NEW BODY: Close your eyes and take a few relaxing breaths—in through your nose and out through your mouth. Visualize that you are standing in a dressing room and can see every angle of your body in the mirrors. Now I want you to look at the body you have worked so hard to build. Starting from the tip of your head, scan all the way down to the bottom of your feet. What do you see? Do you like what you see? Look at your face and how smooth and taut your skin looks. Look at your neck and notice the lack of sagging skin. Now look at your shoulders and see how strong and defined they are. The 12-Second Sequence™ has made your arms toned and so strong. Look at how lean and tight your tummy is. Look down at your thighs, how lean and defined the muscles are. Stretch your leg out and watch as the muscles contract, all the way down your leg. Beautiful! Look in the mirror behind you and see your strong back. Where there used to be love handles, there are now smooth, lean muscles. Keep looking in the mirror at your new body for as long as you like.

DATE: _____

EATING PLANNER

This plan will ensure leaner muscle and a higher metabolism.

Breakfast>time_____   Description

		Description
○	PROTEIN* (3–5oz/40g)	
○	CARBS (½ cup or 1 slice of bread)	
○	FRUIT (1 cup)	
○	FAT (1 teaspoon)	

Snack>time_____   Description

		Description
○	WHEY PROTEIN SHAKE (1 scoop)	

Jorge recommends Jorge's Packs™ protein drinks. > See other recommended snacks at the back of the journal.

Lunch>time_____   Description

		Description
○	PROTEIN* (3–5oz/40g)	
○	CARBS (½ cup or 1 slice of bread)	
○	VEGGIES** (2 cups)	
○	FAT (1 teaspoon)	

Snack>time_____   Description

		Description
○	WHEY PROTEIN SHAKE (1 scoop)	

Dinner>time_____   Description

		Description
○	PROTEIN* (3–5oz/40g)	
○	VEGGIES** (2–4 cups)	
○	FAT (1 teaspoon)	

Snack>time_____   Description

		Description
○	WHEY PROTEIN SHAKE (1 scoop)	

*If you weigh under 150 pounds, eat 3 ounces of protein at every meal; if you weigh over 150 pounds, eat 5 ounces of protein.

**Veggies = nonstarchy vegetables.

Water (eight 8-oz cups) ○ ○ ○ ○ ○ ○ ○ ○

Multivitamin ○

WORKOUT LOG   WEEK_____ OF 8

Primary Workout

DATE_____ DAY_____ OF 56

Start>time_____ Finish>time_____

TOTAL TIME_____

Select weights so that by the end of the fourth rep of each exercise you feel an intensity level of 8.

	Muscle Group	Exercise	Weight Used	Intensity Level
CIRCUIT 1	LEGS			
	BACK			
	CHEST			
	ABS			

At this point you should be about 6 minutes into your workout.

	Muscle Group	Exercise	Weight Used	Intensity Level
CIRCUIT 2	LEGS			
	BACK			
	CHEST			
	ABS			

At this point you should be about 14 minutes into your workout, including 2 minutes of transition time.

	Muscle Group	Exercise	Weight Used	Intensity Level
CIRCUIT 3	LEGS			
	BACK			
	CHEST			
	ABS			

At this point in your workout you should be at 20 minutes. Congratulations! YOU DID IT!

BONUS CARDIO 26-MINUTE MORNING POWER WALK ○

After my workout I feel _____

(e.g., confident, strong)

< REFLECTIONS >

> > > **Above all, challenge yourself. You may well surprise yourself at what strengths you have, what you can accomplish.**

—CECILE SPRINGER

Day Off! > NO WORKOUT TODAY

REFLECTIONS _____

_____

_____

_____

Jorge's Meditation > EMBRACE YOUR NATURAL GIFTS: If your time and money were unlimited, and you could do anything in the world that you wanted to do, what would it be? To help you come up with your answer, think about your natural gifts. To unlock the secrets behind your special gifts, take a moment to step back and look at yourself through the eyes of those who love you. What have they told you that they believe are your special gifts? Now, look closely at yourself and do an assessment of your strengths and weaknesses. What can you do to develop your weaknesses into strengths? Next, list your opportunities. Look at what strengths you possess in terms of talents; using these natural gifts will bring joy into your life.

BONUS CARDIO 26-MINUTE MORNING POWER WALK ○

DATE:

EATING PLANNER

This plan will ensure leaner muscle and a higher metabolism.

Breakfast>time_____   Description

○	PROTEIN* (3–5oz/40g)	
○	CARBS (½ cup or 1 slice of bread)	
○	FRUIT (1 cup)	
○	FAT (1 teaspoon)	

Snack>time_____   Description

○	WHEY PROTEIN SHAKE (1 scoop)	

Jorge recommends Jorge's Packs™ protein drinks. > See other recommended snacks at the back of the journal.

Lunch>time_____   Description

○	PROTEIN* (3–5oz/40g)	
○	CARBS (½ cup or 1 slice of bread)	
○	VEGGIES** (2 cups)	
○	FAT (1 teaspoon)	

Snack>time_____   Description

○	WHEY PROTEIN SHAKE (1 scoop)	

Dinner>time_____   Description

○	PROTEIN* (3–5oz/40g)	
○	VEGGIES** (2–4 cups)	
○	FAT (1 teaspoon)	

Snack>time_____   Description

○	WHEY PROTEIN SHAKE (1 scoop)	

*If you weigh under 150 pounds, eat 3 ounces of protein at every meal; if you weigh over 150 pounds, eat 5 ounces of protein.

**Veggies = nonstarchy vegetables.

Water (eight 8-oz cups) ○ ○ ○ ○ ○ ○ ○ ○

Multivitamin ○

> > > The first wealth is health. —RALPH WALDO EMERSON

Day Off! > NO WORKOUT TODAY

REFLECTIONS _____

_____

_____

_____

_____

Jorge's Meditation > THE RIGHT KIND OF STRESS: Wouldn't it be great to get rid of all the stress in your life? Well . . . not exactly. There are actually two different kinds of stress: *eustress,* which is good stress, and *distress,* which is the type of stress that causes us to feel powerless in overwhelming situations. Eustress motivates us and enhances our successes in life. Distress often leads us to overeat, slack off on our workouts, or develop other self-destructive behaviors. The first step in dealing with distress is to understand which situations stress you out. Create a list of the people, places, and events that make your body react negatively, and how your body reacts to these situations. Once you identify your stressors, you're ready to conquer them. Do a visualization exercise before you enter one of these situations and envision yourself staying calm and relaxed. If you feel stress coming on, take a moment to relax, do a deep-breathing exercise, and bring your attention inward to focus your mind on your body and calming it down. When you know how to control your body and read the signals of distress, you can change the energy of the situation and turn it into eustress.

BONUS CARDIO 26-MINUTE MORNING POWER WALK ○

DATE: _____

EATING PLANNER

This plan will ensure leaner muscle and a higher metabolism.

Breakfast>time_____   Description

○	PROTEIN* (3–5oz/40g)	
○	CARBS (½ cup or 1 slice of bread)	
○	FRUIT (1 cup)	
○	FAT (1 teaspoon)	

Snack>time_____   Description

| ○ | WHEY PROTEIN SHAKE (1 scoop) | |

Jorge recommends Jorge's Packs™ protein drinks. **>** See other recommended snacks at the back of the journal.

Lunch>time_____   Description

○	PROTEIN* (3–5oz/40g)	
○	CARBS (½ cup or 1 slice of bread)	
○	VEGGIES** (2 cups)	
○	FAT (1 teaspoon)	

Snack>time_____   Description

| ○ | WHEY PROTEIN SHAKE (1 scoop) | |

Dinner>time_____   Description

○	PROTEIN* (3–5oz/40g)	
○	VEGGIES** (2–4 cups)	
○	FAT (1 teaspoon)	

Snack>time_____   Description

| ○ | WHEY PROTEIN SHAKE (1 scoop) | |

*If you weigh under 150 pounds, eat 3 ounces of protein at every meal; if you weigh over 150 pounds, eat 5 ounces of protein.

**Veggies = nonstarchy vegetables.

Water (eight 8-oz cups) ○ ○ ○ ○ ○ ○ ○ ○
Multivitamin ○

> > > **There's only one way to succeed in anything, and that is to give it every-thing.** —VINCE LOMBARDI

Jorge's Meditation > YOUR DREAM VACATION: Close your eyes and take a few relaxing breaths—in through your nose and out through your mouth. Visualize yourself on an airplane, stretched out in a roomy first-class seat. As you gaze out the window at the crystal-blue water below, the captain's voice comes over the intercom: "I hope everyone had a pleasant flight. The current temperature in Maui is a pleasant 78 degrees and there's not a cloud in the sky." You collect your suitcases at the baggage claim and hop into a taxi to go to your hotel. Imagine the gorgeous scenery whipping by you as you drive along. When you arrive at your hotel, you're greeted by a hula girl who places a beautiful orchid lei around your neck. When you get to your hotel room, you head straight to your balcony and take a deep breath in and look out at the white sandy beach. You listen to the waves as they crash on shore and think about how far you've come to get to this point in your life. Your hard work and determination have really paid off. So with a whole week in paradise ahead of you, think about what activities you'll be doing. Have a great vacation. You deserve it!

DATE:

EATING PLANNER

This plan will ensure leaner muscle and a higher metabolism.

Breakfast>time_____
Description

○	PROTEIN* (3–5oz/40g)	
○	CARBS (½ cup or 1 slice of bread)	
○	FRUIT (1 cup)	
○	FAT (1 teaspoon)	

Snack>time_____
Description

○	WHEY PROTEIN SHAKE (1 scoop)	

Jorge recommends Jorge's Packs™ protein drinks. **>** See other recommended snacks at the back of the journal.

Lunch>time_____
Description

○	PROTEIN* (3–5oz/40g)	
○	CARBS (½ cup or 1 slice of bread)	
○	VEGGIES** (2 cups)	
○	FAT (1 teaspoon)	

Snack>time_____
Description

○	WHEY PROTEIN SHAKE (1 scoop)	

Dinner>time_____
Description

○	PROTEIN* (3–5oz/40g)	
○	VEGGIES** (2–4 cups)	
○	FAT (1 teaspoon)	

Snack>time_____
Description

○	WHEY PROTEIN SHAKE (1 scoop)	

*If you weigh under 150 pounds, eat 3 ounces of protein at every meal; if you weigh over 150 pounds, eat 5 ounces of protein.

**Veggies = nonstarchy vegetables.

Water (eight 8-oz cups) ○ ○ ○ ○ ○ ○ ○ ○

Multivitamin ○

WORKOUT LOG

WEEK_____OF 8

Secondary Workout

DATE_____ DAY _____ OF 56

Start>time_____ Finish>time_____

TOTAL TIME_____

Select weights so that by the end of the fourth rep of each exercise you feel an intensity level of 8.

Muscle Group	Exercise	Weight Used	Intensity Level
CIRCUIT 1			
SHOULDERS			
BICEPS			
TRICEPS			
ABS			

At this point you should be about 6 minutes into your workout.

Muscle Group	Exercise	Weight Used	Intensity Level
CIRCUIT 2			
SHOULDERS			
BICEPS			
TRICEPS			
ABS			

At this point you should be about 14 minutes into your workout, including 2 minutes of transition time.

Muscle Group	Exercise	Weight Used	Intensity Level
CIRCUIT 3			
SHOULDERS			
BICEPS			
TRICEPS			
ABS			

At this point in your workout you should be at 20 minutes. Congratulations! YOU DID IT!

BONUS CARDIO 26-MINUTE MORNING POWER WALK ○

After my workout I feel_____

(e.g., confident, strong)

< REFLECTIONS >

> > > **If you don't do what's best for your body, you're the one who comes up on the short end.** —JULIUS ERVING

Day Off! > NO WORKOUT TODAY

REFLECTIONS _____

_____

_____

_____

Jorge's Meditation > EATING SMART: I love to eat. When I lost weight and got fit, I learned that you don't have to give up your favorite foods or feel deprived to stay slim and shapely. Here's a great trick I learned that might help you eat fewer of the calories on your plate and still enjoy dining with your family and friends. Look at your plate and pick out the lowest-calorie food on it. Most typically it will be your veggie portion. So go ahead and eat your veggies to fill you up. After that, pick out the next-lowest-calorie item on your plate and eat it up, and so on and so on. Save the highest-calorie item for last, and you might surprise yourself—you'll probably be too full to finish it! Now, if this trick doesn't work for you and you tend to keep eating because you left your favorite food for last, no problem—just reverse the order. Eat your favorite foods first so you have less room for the calories you don't care about. Bottom line: think about what you're eating and make each bite of it enjoyable and worthwhile.

BONUS CARDIO 26-MINUTE MORNING POWER WALK ○

DATE: _____

EATING PLANNER

This plan will ensure leaner muscle and a higher metabolism.

Breakfast>time_____   Description

○ PROTEIN* (3–5oz/40g)	
○ CARBS (½ cup or 1 slice of bread)	
○ FRUIT (1 cup)	
○ FAT (1 teaspoon)	

Snack>time_____   Description

○ WHEY PROTEIN SHAKE (1 scoop)	

Jorge recommends Jorge's Packs™ protein drinks. **>** See other recommended snacks at the back of the journal.

Lunch>time_____   Description

○ PROTEIN* (3–5oz/40g)	
○ CARBS (½ cup or 1 slice of bread)	
○ VEGGIES** (2 cups)	
○ FAT (1 teaspoon)	

Snack>time_____   Description

○ WHEY PROTEIN SHAKE (1 scoop)	

Dinner>time_____   Description

○ PROTEIN* (3–5oz/40g)	
○ VEGGIES** (2–4 cups)	
○ FAT (1 teaspoon)	

Snack>time_____   Description

○ WHEY PROTEIN SHAKE (1 scoop)	

*If you weigh under 150 pounds, eat 3 ounces of protein at every meal; if you weigh over 150 pounds, eat 5 ounces of protein.

**Veggies = nonstarchy vegetables.

Water (eight 8-oz cups) ○ ○ ○ ○ ○ ○ ○ ○

Multivitamin ○

> > > **If you hear a voice within you say "you cannot paint," by all means paint, and that voice will be silenced.** —VINCENT VAN GOGH

Day Off! > NO WORKOUT TODAY

REFLECTIONS _____

_____

_____

_____

_____

Jorge's Meditation > WALK YOUR WAY TO FITNESS: A pedometer looks like a beeper and clips onto your waistband, or hangs from your neck. It may be one of the most effective electronic tools for weight loss, fitness, and health. Remember, strength training is the smartest way to lose weight, but by incorporating more walking into your day, you can tap into quick "bonus" calories. A pedometer provides great motivation. We can all tell ourselves to park farther away from the grocery store or take the stairs rather than the elevator, but when you wear a pedometer, you can look down and see that all those steps really do add up. Write down in this journal every night the total number of steps you took and set goals that will encourage you to take a few more steps every day.

BONUS CARDIO 26-MINUTE MORNING POWER WALK ○

DATE:

EATING PLANNER

This plan will ensure leaner muscle and a higher metabolism.

Breakfast>time_____

Description

○ PROTEIN* (3–5oz/40g)	
○ CARBS (½ cup or 1 slice of bread)	
○ FRUIT (1 cup)	
○ FAT (1 teaspoon)	

Snack>time_____

Description

○ WHEY PROTEIN SHAKE (1 scoop)	

Jorge recommends Jorge's Packs™ protein drinks. **>** See other recommended snacks at the back of the journal.

Lunch>time_____

Description

○ PROTEIN* (3–5oz/40g)	
○ CARBS (½ cup or 1 slice of bread)	
○ VEGGIES** (2 cups)	
○ FAT (1 teaspoon)	

Snack>time_____

Description

○ WHEY PROTEIN SHAKE (1 scoop)	

Dinner>time_____

Description

○ PROTEIN* (3–5oz/40g)	
○ VEGGIES** (2–4 cups)	
○ FAT (1 teaspoon)	

Snack>time_____

Description

○ WHEY PROTEIN SHAKE (1 scoop)	

*If you weigh under 150 pounds, eat 3 ounces of protein at every meal; if you weigh over 150 pounds, eat 5 ounces of protein.

**Veggies = nonstarchy vegetables.

Water (eight 8-oz cups) ○ ○ ○ ○ ○ ○ ○ ○

Multivitamin ○

> > > **Great works are performed, not by strength, but by perseverance.**

—SAMUEL JOHNSON

Day Off! > NO WORKOUT TODAY

REFLECTIONS _____

_____

_____

_____

Jorge's Meditation > TIMING: You know that timing is an important component of success in the 12-Second Sequence™. You need to count the 10-second positive motion, the 2-second static hold, and the 10-second negative motion. If you count too slowly, you'll extend your workout beyond 20 minutes; if you count too quickly, you won't fully saturate your muscles and you'll miss out on getting the full impact of your workout. But how do you count accurately when you're concentrating on so many other things, like form and breathing? I like to use a metronome. A metronome is a simple device that musicians use to help them keep time. Whether you use a metronome or simply count on your own, remember that each second matters in the 12-Second Sequence™. Don't cheat yourself; make your workout time worthwhile.

BONUS CARDIO 26-MINUTE MORNING POWER WALK ○

DATE:

EATING PLANNER

This plan will ensure leaner muscle and a higher metabolism.

Breakfast>time_____   Description

○	**PROTEIN*** (3–5oz/40g)	
○	**CARBS** (½ cup or 1 slice of bread)	
○	**FRUIT** (1 cup)	
○	**FAT** (1 teaspoon)	

Snack>time_____   Description

○	**WHEY PROTEIN SHAKE** (1 scoop)

Jorge recommends Jorge's Packs™ protein drinks. **>** See other recommended snacks at the back of the journal.

Lunch>time_____   Description

○	**PROTEIN*** (3–5oz/40g)	
○	**CARBS** (½ cup or 1 slice of bread)	
○	**VEGGIES**** (2 cups)	
○	**FAT** (1 teaspoon)	

Snack>time_____   Description

○	**WHEY PROTEIN SHAKE** (1 scoop)

Dinner>time_____   Description

○	**PROTEIN*** (3–5oz/40g)	
○	**VEGGIES**** (2–4 cups)	
○	**FAT** (1 teaspoon)	

Snack>time_____   Description

○	**WHEY PROTEIN SHAKE** (1 scoop)

*If you weigh under 150 pounds, eat 3 ounces of protein at every meal; if you weigh over 150 pounds, eat 5 ounces of protein.

**Veggies = nonstarchy vegetables.

Water (eight 8-oz cups) ○ ○ ○ ○ ○ ○ ○ ○

Multivitamin ○

> > > **Twenty years from now you will be more disappointed by the things you didn't do than by the ones you did do.** —MARK TWAIN

Jorge's Meditation > SEE THE FUTURE YOU: Close your eyes and take a few deep, relaxing breaths—in through your nose and out through your mouth. Imagine you are seated in a huge auditorium filled with your friends and family, the media, fitness professionals, and people who are looking for inspiration to get in shape. The presenter takes the stage, introduces himself, and begins to tell the audience about a very special person who has come a long way. Your before picture is projected on a screen behind the presenter and you look up at your former self. The presenter speaks: "Ladies and gentlemen, it is truly an honor to present [your name] with the Dynamic Achievement Award for healthy living. She has come a long way from the picture behind me and she is an inspiration to us all. And here she is . . ." As thunderous applause shakes the auditorium and an orchestra plays, you stride to the stage. You take the award in your hands and the audience quiets down to hear you speak. What do you say into the microphone? After your final words, the auditorium again booms with applause and you look out at the standing ovation.

DATE:

EATING PLANNER

This plan will ensure leaner muscle and a higher metabolism.

Breakfast>time_____   Description

○	PROTEIN* (3–5oz/40g)	
○	CARBS (½ cup or 1 slice of bread)	
○	FRUIT (1 cup)	
○	FAT (1 teaspoon)	

Snack>time_____   Description

○	WHEY PROTEIN SHAKE (1 scoop)

Jorge recommends Jorge's Packs™ protein drinks. > See other recommended snacks at the back of the journal.

Lunch>time_____   Description

○	PROTEIN* (3–5oz/40g)	
○	CARBS (½ cup or 1 slice of bread)	
○	VEGGIES** (2 cups)	
○	FAT (1 teaspoon)	

Snack>time_____   Description

○	WHEY PROTEIN SHAKE (1 scoop)

Dinner>time_____   Description

○	PROTEIN* (3–5oz/40g)	
○	VEGGIES** (2–4 cups)	
○	FAT (1 teaspoon)	

Snack>time_____   Description

○	WHEY PROTEIN SHAKE (1 scoop)

*If you weigh under 150 pounds, eat 3 ounces of protein at every meal; if you weigh over 150 pounds, eat 5 ounces of protein.

**Veggies = nonstarchy vegetables.

Water (eight 8-oz cups) ○ ○ ○ ○ ○ ○ ○ ○

Multivitamin ○

WORKOUT LOG | WEEK_____ OF 8

Primary Workout

DATE_____ DAY_____ OF 56

Start>time_____ Finish>time_____

TOTAL TIME_____

Select weights so that by the end of the fourth rep of each exercise you feel an intensity level of 8.

	Muscle Group	Exercise	Weight Used	Intensity Level
CIRCUIT 1	LEGS			
	BACK			
	CHEST			
	ABS			

At this point you should be about 6 minutes into your workout.

	Muscle Group	Exercise	Weight Used	Intensity Level
CIRCUIT 2	LEGS			
	BACK			
	CHEST			
	ABS			

At this point you should be about 14 minutes into your workout, including 2 minutes of transition time.

	Muscle Group	Exercise	Weight Used	Intensity Level
CIRCUIT 3	LEGS			
	BACK			
	CHEST			
	ABS			

At this point in your workout you should be at 20 minutes. Congratulations! YOU DID IT!

BONUS CARDIO 26-MINUTE MORNING POWER WALK ○

After my workout I feel_____

(e.g., confident, strong)

< REFLECTIONS >

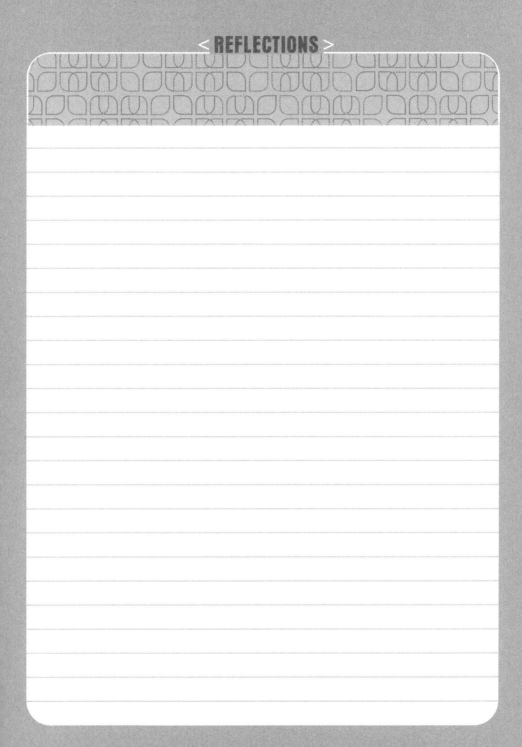

> > > **Health, learning and virtue will ensure your happiness.** —THOMAS JEFFERSON

Day Off! > NO WORKOUT TODAY

REFLECTIONS

_____

_____

_____

_____

Jorge's Meditation > LOSE YOUR LOSER ZONE: All of us have what I call the Loser Zone. It's where most of us spend much of our free time. You're in a Loser Zone when you're doing something that produces no significant improvement in your life. The number one Loser Zone activity is watching television. Did you know that the average American spends thirty hours a week watching TV? Another Loser Zone activity is playing video games or aimlessly surfing the Net. When participating in these activities, time speeds out of our grasp; we're "zoned out." Fight back! You can regain your free time by recognizing your Loser Zones and limiting how much time you spend in them. If watching TV is your biggest Loser Zone, limit yourself to watching only the show you want to watch and then turning it off after the show is over. You can also try using an alarm clock or kitchen timer to regulate how much time you spend in your Loser Zones. With all that newly found time, do something great for your body and soul!

BONUS CARDIO 26-MINUTE MORNING POWER WALK ○

DATE:

EATING PLANNER

This plan will ensure leaner muscle and a higher metabolism.

Breakfast>time_____   Description

○	PROTEIN* (3–5oz/40g)	
○	CARBS (½ cup or 1 slice of bread)	
○	FRUIT (1 cup)	
○	FAT (1 teaspoon)	

Snack>time_____   Description

○	WHEY PROTEIN SHAKE (1 scoop)	

Jorge recommends Jorge's Packs™ protein drinks. **>** See other recommended snacks at the back of the journal.

Lunch>time_____   Description

○	PROTEIN* (3–5oz/40g)	
○	CARBS (½ cup or 1 slice of bread)	
○	VEGGIES** (2 cups)	
○	FAT (1 teaspoon)	

Snack>time_____   Description

○	WHEY PROTEIN SHAKE (1 scoop)	

Dinner>time_____   Description

○	PROTEIN* (3–5oz/40g)	
○	VEGGIES** (2–4 cups)	
○	FAT (1 teaspoon)	

Snack>time_____   Description

○	WHEY PROTEIN SHAKE (1 scoop)	

*If you weigh under 150 pounds, eat 3 ounces of protein at every meal; if you weigh over 150 pounds, eat 5 ounces of protein.

**Veggies = nonstarchy vegetables.

Water (eight 8-oz cups) ○ ○ ○ ○ ○ ○ ○ ○

Multivitamin ○

> > > **What would you attempt to do if you knew you could not fail?**

—ROBERT SCHULLER

Day Off! > NO WORKOUT TODAY

REFLECTIONS _____

_____

_____

_____

Jorge's Meditation > PUSH VS. PULL: Many very successful people achieved great things by focusing on what they were passionate about. Bill Gates, for example, didn't set out to become the richest man in America. His goal was, and still is, to find something new every day. Chasing that goal enabled him to become extraordinarily successful—while doing something he loved. That's a huge key to success—finding something that is so compelling, so fulfilling, that it pulls you toward your goal instead of pushing you. When you have to push yourself, it's tough to get up and walk every morning and stick to a healthy diet every day. Pushing yourself makes these everyday tasks seem harder and makes your ultimate goal seem farther and farther away. However, when you think about what you're working toward—a healthy, beautiful body and a longer, better-quality life—your goal pulls you to accomplish these daily milestones. You're inspired, not forced, to stick to your diet, work out twice a week, and walk every day. It becomes automatic.

BONUS CARDIO 26-MINUTE MORNING POWER WALK ○

DATE:

EATING PLANNER

This plan will ensure leaner muscle and a higher metabolism.

Breakfast>time_____   Description

○	PROTEIN* (3–5oz/40g)	
○	CARBS (½ cup or 1 slice of bread)	
○	FRUIT (1 cup)	
○	FAT (1 teaspoon)	

Snack>time_____   Description

○	WHEY PROTEIN SHAKE (1 scoop)	

Jorge recommends Jorge's Packs™ protein drinks. **>** See other recommended snacks at the back of the journal.

Lunch>time_____   Description

○	PROTEIN* (3–5oz/40g)	
○	CARBS (½ cup or 1 slice of bread)	
○	VEGGIES** (2 cups)	
○	FAT (1 teaspoon)	

Snack>time_____   Description

○	WHEY PROTEIN SHAKE (1 scoop)	

Dinner>time_____   Description

○	PROTEIN* (3–5oz/40g)	
○	VEGGIES** (2–4 cups)	
○	FAT (1 teaspoon)	

Snack>time_____   Description

○	WHEY PROTEIN SHAKE (1 scoop)	

*If you weigh under 150 pounds, eat 3 ounces of protein at every meal; if you weigh over 150 pounds,
  eat 5 ounces of protein.

**Veggies = nonstarchy vegetables.

Water (eight 8-oz cups) ○ ○ ○ ○ ○ ○ ○ ○

Multivitamin ○

> > > **The higher your energy level, the more efficient your body. The more efficient your body, the better you feel and the more you will use your talent to produce outstanding results.**

—ANTHONY ROBBINS

Jorge's Meditation > CREATE YOUR OWN LUCK: Anyone can catch the magic of their "lucky stars" and make things go their way simply by having a goal, creating the vision, and thinking positively. Determining and setting your goal is the first critical step in making your own luck. The moment you fully commit to a goal is the moment that goal becomes a reality. Without full commitment, a goal is just a goal; it's like an empty pot at the end of the rainbow. By setting the date you will achieve your goal weight, and also the dates for your mini goals, you are essentially putting the gold in the pot. To follow the rainbow to your pot of gold, or better yet, pot of goals, you must next figure out what the rainbow looks like. By creating a clear picture of your future body at your goal weight you are making your own luck; you are able to see, touch, taste, and feel the rainbow that leads to your goals. Remember, you create your own luck.

DATE:

EATING PLANNER
This plan will ensure leaner muscle and a higher metabolism.

Breakfast>time_____   Description

○	**PROTEIN*** (3–5oz/40g)	
○	**CARBS** (½ cup or 1 slice of bread)	
○	**FRUIT** (1 cup)	
○	**FAT** (1 teaspoon)	

Snack>time_____   Description

○	**WHEY PROTEIN SHAKE** (1 scoop)	

Jorge recommends Jorge's Packs™ protein drinks. **>** See other recommended snacks at the back of the journal.

Lunch>time_____   Description

○	**PROTEIN*** (3–5oz/40g)	
○	**CARBS** (½ cup or 1 slice of bread)	
○	**VEGGIES**** (2 cups)	
○	**FAT** (1 teaspoon)	

Snack>time_____   Description

○	**WHEY PROTEIN SHAKE** (1 scoop)	

Dinner>time_____   Description

○	**PROTEIN*** (3–5oz/40g)	
○	**VEGGIES**** (2–4 cups)	
○	**FAT** (1 teaspoon)	

Snack>time_____   Description

○	**WHEY PROTEIN SHAKE** (1 scoop)	

*If you weigh under 150 pounds, eat 3 ounces of protein at every meal; if you weigh over 150 pounds, eat 5 ounces of protein.

**Veggies = nonstarchy vegetables.

Water (eight 8-oz cups) ○ ○ ○ ○ ○ ○ ○ ○

Multivitamin ○

WORKOUT LOG WEEK____OF 8

Secondary Workout

DATE_____ DAY____ OF 56

Start>time_____ Finish>time_____

TOTAL TIME_____

Select weights so that by the end of the fourth rep of each exercise you feel an intensity level of 8.

Muscle Group	Exercise	Weight Used	Intensity Level
CIRCUIT 1			
SHOULDERS			
BICEPS			
TRICEPS			
ABS			

At this point you should be about 6 minutes into your workout.

Muscle Group	Exercise	Weight Used	Intensity Level
CIRCUIT 2			
SHOULDERS			
BICEPS			
TRICEPS			
ABS			

At this point you should be about 14 minutes into your workout, including 2 minutes of transition time.

Muscle Group	Exercise	Weight Used	Intensity Level
CIRCUIT 3			
SHOULDERS			
BICEPS			
TRICEPS			
ABS			

At this point in your workout you should be at 20 minutes. Congratulations! YOU DID IT!

BONUS CARDIO 26-MINUTE MORNING POWER WALK ○

After my workout I feel_____

(e.g., confident, strong)

< REFLECTIONS >

> > > **Your goals, minus your doubts, equal your reality.** —RALPH MARSTON

Day Off! > **NO WORKOUT TODAY**

REFLECTIONS _____

_____

_____

_____

Jorge's Meditation > RELISH EVERY MOMENT: So many people walk through life on auto pilot and don't pay attention to their everyday actions. Once you become cognizant of your patterns and begin to see yourself objectively, you can get back in touch with who you really are and make changes that will help you get what you really want out of life. To become aware of your life, try to observe and remember what you are doing at every moment of the day—become conscious of everything! When you get into the habit of noticing and thinking about your actions and feelings, you will be able to discover which situations make you react in certain ways and what needs to be changed. Lessons will be repeated until learned and the only way to learn them is to become aware. Before you fall asleep at night, ask yourself "What did I do today?" and make your answer so lengthy that you've fallen sound asleep before you've thought about it all. Your days are yours to live and learn from, so become aware and relish every moment.

BONUS CARDIO 26-MINUTE MORNING POWER WALK ○

DATE:

EATING PLANNER

This plan will ensure leaner muscle and a higher metabolism.

Breakfast>time_____   Description

○	PROTEIN* (3–5oz/40g)	
○	CARBS (½ cup or 1 slice of bread)	
○	FRUIT (1 cup)	
○	FAT (1 teaspoon)	

Snack>time_____   Description

○	WHEY PROTEIN SHAKE (1 scoop)	

Jorge recommends Jorge's Packs™ protein drinks. **>** See other recommended snacks at the back of the journal.

Lunch>time_____   Description

○	PROTEIN* (3–5oz/40g)	
○	CARBS (½ cup or 1 slice of bread)	
○	VEGGIES** (2 cups)	
○	FAT (1 teaspoon)	

Snack>time_____   Description

○	WHEY PROTEIN SHAKE (1 scoop)	

Dinner>time_____   Description

○	PROTEIN* (3–5oz/40g)	
○	VEGGIES** (2–4 cups)	
○	FAT (1 teaspoon)	

Snack>time_____   Description

○	WHEY PROTEIN SHAKE (1 scoop)	

*If you weigh under 150 pounds, eat 3 ounces of protein at every meal; if you weigh over 150 pounds, eat 5 ounces of protein.

**Veggies = nonstarchy vegetables.

Water (eight 8-oz cups) ○ ○ ○ ○ ○ ○ ○ ○
Multivitamin ○

> > > **We can do anything we want to if we stick to it long enough.** —HELEN KELLER

Day Off! > NO WORKOUT TODAY

REFLECTIONS

_____

_____

_____

_____

Jorge's Meditation > **POWER LABELS:** Too many people unconsciously label themselves in ways that make them feel bad: over the hill, overeater, couch potato, lazy . . . the list could go on. Even though you might think these labels are innocent, the human brain is such a powerful instrument that you will eventually become whatever you label yourself. Even though it is just a saying, it will become real when you take it on. To achieve your best body ever, I want you to create a new, positive Power Label for yourself that will get you excited about exercising and eating well. Some examples of motivating Power Labels are _superwoman, superman,_ and _athlete._ Make up something that works for you and remind yourself of it throughout the day. Another trick that will help you jump-start your motivation is to use empowering metaphors. Words and phrases can powerfully and instantly affect how you feel about things, and using power metaphors will help keep you motivated to get lean. Here are some examples, but try to make up some on your own as well: "Food is fuel." "Life is a game." "Food is my medicine." "Exercise is a gift."

BONUS CARDIO 26-MINUTE MORNING POWER WALK ○

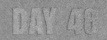

DATE:

EATING PLANNER
This plan will ensure leaner muscle and a higher metabolism.

Breakfast>time_____   Description

○	PROTEIN* (3–5oz/40g)	
○	CARBS (½ cup or 1 slice of bread)	
○	FRUIT (1 cup)	
○	FAT (1 teaspoon)	

Snack>time_____   Description

○	WHEY PROTEIN SHAKE (1 scoop)	

Jorge recommends Jorge's Packs™ protein drinks. **>** See other recommended snacks at the back of the journal.

Lunch>time_____   Description

○	PROTEIN* (3–5oz/40g)	
○	CARBS (½ cup or 1 slice of bread)	
○	VEGGIES** (2 cups)	
○	FAT (1 teaspoon)	

Snack>time_____   Description

○	WHEY PROTEIN SHAKE (1 scoop)	

Dinner>time_____   Description

○	PROTEIN* (3–5oz/40g)	
○	VEGGIES** (2–4 cups)	
○	FAT (1 teaspoon)	

Snack>time_____   Description

○	WHEY PROTEIN SHAKE (1 scoop)	

*If you weigh under 150 pounds, eat 3 ounces of protein at every meal; if you weigh over 150 pounds,
  eat 5 ounces of protein.

**Veggies = nonstarchy vegetables.

Water (eight 8-oz cups) ○ ○ ○ ○ ○ ○ ○ ○

Multivitamin ○

> > > Give your dreams all you've got and you'll be amazed at the energy that comes out of you.

—WILLIAM JAMES

Day Off! > **NO WORKOUT TODAY**

REFLECTIONS _____
_____
_____
_____

Jorge's Meditation > **VISUALIZE YOUR WAY TO SUCCESS:** For these visualization exercises to be the most effective, you need to draw on all of your senses—touch, taste, smell, sight, and sound—as well as how your body feels. The more senses you involve in your visualizations, the more powerful your images will be in making your dreams come true. It's a skill that can be learned and strengthened with practice, so if at first you can't see, feel, taste, smell, or hear the entire scene in the visualization exercises that I take you through, slow down and work on imaging just the very beginning of the scenario, like waking up, and prompt yourself with more detailed questions. How does the pillow feel under your head? What is the first thing that you see as you open your eyes? The more vivid the images, the sooner you'll see and feel the new you begin to emerge.

BONUS CARDIO 26-MINUTE MORNING POWER WALK ○

DATE:

EATING PLANNER

This plan will ensure leaner muscle and a higher metabolism.

Breakfast>time_____   Description

		Description
○	PROTEIN* (3–5oz/40g)	
○	CARBS (½ cup or 1 slice of bread)	
○	FRUIT (1 cup)	
○	FAT (1 teaspoon)	

Snack>time_____   Description

		Description
○	WHEY PROTEIN SHAKE (1 scoop)	

Jorge recommends Jorge's Packs™ protein drinks. **>** See other recommended snacks at the back of the journal.

Lunch>time_____   Description

		Description
○	PROTEIN* (3–5oz/40g)	
○	CARBS (½ cup or 1 slice of bread)	
○	VEGGIES** (2 cups)	
○	FAT (1 teaspoon)	

Snack>time_____   Description

		Description
○	WHEY PROTEIN SHAKE (1 scoop)	

Dinner>time_____   Description

		Description
○	PROTEIN* (3–5oz/40g)	
○	VEGGIES** (2–4 cups)	
○	FAT (1 teaspoon)	

Snack>time_____   Description

		Description
○	WHEY PROTEIN SHAKE (1 scoop)	

*If you weigh under 150 pounds, eat 3 ounces of protein at every meal; if you weigh over 150 pounds, eat 5 ounces of protein.

**Veggies = nonstarchy vegetables.

Water (eight 8-oz cups) ○ ○ ○ ○ ○ ○ ○ ○

Multivitamin ○

> > > **Why wait? Life is not a dress rehearsal. Quit practicing what you're going to do, and just do it. In one bold stroke you can transform today.** —MARILYN GREY

Jorge's Meditation > WE'RE ALL HUMAN: We all have days when our best-laid plans go awry. However, we do have the power to change how we react. Let's say you find yourself at your office party and one bite of cake leads to another and another, and the next thing you know, you've swallowed the equivalent of what you'd normally eat in a couple of days. Don't beat yourself up about it; you must have the generosity and wisdom to forgive yourself. One of the biggest mistakes people make when they're trying to get in shape is that they don't accept their slipups, which leads them to chuck the whole thing, disregarding past successes and throwing aside future victories. But setbacks aren't the end of a weight-loss effort; they are a part of the process and your ability to change for the better is only enhanced by experiences—both good and bad. You must learn from your mistakes and adjust for future success. Write about the situation in this journal. Talk about it with your buddy team. You can learn, you can grow, and you can become more and more of what you want to be.

DATE: _____

EATING PLANNER

This plan will ensure leaner muscle and a higher metabolism.

Breakfast>time_____   Description

	Description
○ PROTEIN* (3–5oz/40g)	
○ CARBS (½ cup or 1 slice of bread)	
○ FRUIT (1 cup)	
○ FAT (1 teaspoon)	

Snack>time_____   Description

○ WHEY PROTEIN SHAKE (1 scoop)	

Jorge recommends Jorge's Packs™ protein drinks. **>** See other recommended snacks at the back of the journal.

Lunch>time_____   Description

	Description
○ PROTEIN* (3–5oz/40g)	
○ CARBS (½ cup or 1 slice of bread)	
○ VEGGIES** (2 cups)	
○ FAT (1 teaspoon)	

Snack>time_____   Description

○ WHEY PROTEIN SHAKE (1 scoop)	

Dinner>time_____   Description

	Description
○ PROTEIN* (3–5oz/40g)	
○ VEGGIES** (2–4 cups)	
○ FAT (1 teaspoon)	

Snack>time_____   Description

○ WHEY PROTEIN SHAKE (1 scoop)	

*If you weigh under 150 pounds, eat 3 ounces of protein at every meal; if you weigh over 150 pounds, eat 5 ounces of protein.

**Veggies = nonstarchy vegetables.

Water (eight 8-oz cups) ○ ○ ○ ○ ○ ○ ○ ○
Multivitamin ○

DAY 50   12-Second Sequence™

Primary Workout

DATE_____ DAY____ OF 56

Start>time_____ Finish>time_____

TOTAL TIME_____

Select weights so that by the end of the fourth rep of each exercise you feel an intensity level of 8.

Muscle Group	Exercise	Weight Used	Intensity Level
CIRCUIT 1			
LEGS			
BACK			
CHEST			
ABS			

At this point you should be about 6 minutes into your workout.

Muscle Group	Exercise	Weight Used	Intensity Level
CIRCUIT 2			
LEGS			
BACK			
CHEST			
ABS			

At this point you should be about 14 minutes into your workout, including 2 minutes of transition time.

Muscle Group	Exercise	Weight Used	Intensity Level
CIRCUIT 3			
LEGS			
BACK			
CHEST			
ABS			

At this point in your workout you should be at 20 minutes. Congratulations! YOU DID IT!

BONUS CARDIO 26-MINUTE MORNING POWER WALK ○

After my workout I feel_____

(e.g., confident, strong)

> > > **Getting my lifelong weight struggle under control has come from a process of treating myself as well as I treat others in every way.**

—OPRAH WINFREY

Day Off! > NO WORKOUT TODAY

REFLECTIONS _____

_____

_____

_____

Jorge's Meditation > **PEACE AND SERENITY:** Meditation can help sharpen your focus on your weight-loss goals and ignite your deepest motivation. Choose a quiet spot where you won't be disturbed or distracted and sit in a comfortable position, keeping good posture. Close your eyes and relax your muscles sequentially from head to feet. Start at your forehead, becoming aware of tension as you breathe in. Let go of any obvious tension as you breathe out. Go through the rest of your body in this way, proceeding down through your eyes, jaws, neck, shoulders, arms, hands, chest, upper back, middle back and midriff, lower back, belly, pelvis, buttocks, thighs, calves, and feet. Now continue breathing naturally. Meditation takes practice and though some of the rewards are immediate, like less tension and stress, others take time, often years, to achieve.

BONUS CARDIO 26-MINUTE MORNING POWER WALK ○

DATE:

EATING PLANNER

This plan will ensure leaner muscle and a higher metabolism.

Breakfast>time_____   Description

○	PROTEIN* (3–5oz/40g)	
○	CARBS (½ cup or 1 slice of bread)	
○	FRUIT (1 cup)	
○	FAT (1 teaspoon)	

Snack>time_____   Description

○	WHEY PROTEIN SHAKE (1 scoop)	

Jorge recommends Jorge's Packs™ protein drinks. **>** See other recommended snacks at the back of the journal.

Lunch>time_____   Description

○	PROTEIN* (3–5oz/40g)	
○	CARBS (½ cup or 1 slice of bread)	
○	VEGGIES** (2 cups)	
○	FAT (1 teaspoon)	

Snack>time_____   Description

○	WHEY PROTEIN SHAKE (1 scoop)	

Dinner>time_____   Description

○	PROTEIN* (3–5oz/40g)	
○	VEGGIES** (2–4 cups)	
○	FAT (1 teaspoon)	

Snack>time_____   Description

○	WHEY PROTEIN SHAKE (1 scoop)	

*If you weigh under 150 pounds, eat 3 ounces of protein at every meal; if you weigh over 150 pounds, eat 5 ounces of protein.

**Veggies = nonstarchy vegetables.

Water (eight 8-oz cups) ○ ○ ○ ○ ○ ○ ○ ○

Multivitamin ○

> > > **Your life changes the moment you make a new, congruent, and committed decision.** —ANTHONY ROBBINS

Day Off! > NO WORKOUT TODAY

REFLECTIONS _____

_____

_____

_____

Jorge's Meditation > PROTECT AGAINST ARTHRITIS: For years, arthritis sufferers were discouraged from exercising for fear it might hurt their joints. Over the past decade, this theory has been kicked to the curb as research has proved how basic strength and flexibility exercises can dramatically improve some of the symptoms of arthritis. The reason strength training helps is that strong muscles cushion the joints, acting as shock absorbers. There is cartilage between our bones that absorbs the shock to the joint that gets past the muscle, but without strong muscles, the cartilage endures more damage and wears out much sooner. This pain can lead to reduced activity and weakened muscles, and even more damage. Arthritis sufferers who have a strength-training program have reported a significant decrease in pain; vast improvements in physical function- ing, like being able to climb stairs and sit and stand more easily; and greater self- esteem and self-confidence. Strength training can do great things for your life!

BONUS CARDIO 26-MINUTE MORNING POWER WALK ○

DATE:

EATING PLANNER

This plan will ensure leaner muscle and a higher metabolism.

Breakfast>time_____   Description

○	PROTEIN* (3–5oz/40g)	
○	CARBS (½ cup or 1 slice of bread)	
○	FRUIT (1 cup)	
○	FAT (1 teaspoon)	

Snack>time_____   Description

○	WHEY PROTEIN SHAKE (1 scoop)	

Jorge recommends Jorge's Packs™ protein drinks. **>** See other recommended snacks at the back of the journal.

Lunch>time_____   Description

○	PROTEIN* (3–5oz/40g)	
○	CARBS (½ cup or 1 slice of bread)	
○	VEGGIES** (2 cups)	
○	FAT (1 teaspoon)	

Snack>time_____   Description

○	WHEY PROTEIN SHAKE (1 scoop)	

Dinner>time_____   Description

○	PROTEIN* (3–5oz/40g)	
○	VEGGIES** (2–4 cups)	
○	FAT (1 teaspoon)	

Snack>time_____   Description

○	WHEY PROTEIN SHAKE (1 scoop)	

*If you weigh under 150 pounds, eat 3 ounces of protein at every meal; if you weigh over 150 pounds, eat 5 ounces of protein.

**Veggies = nonstarchy vegetables.

Water (eight 8-oz cups) ○ ○ ○ ○ ○ ○ ○ ○
Multivitamin ○

> > > **The most important key to achieving great success is to decide upon your goal and launch, get started, take action, move.**

—JOHN WOODEN

Jorge's Meditation > A DAY OF SUMMER SHOPPING: Close your eyes and take a few relaxing breaths—in through your nose and out through your mouth. Imagine you're in your car driving to the mall with your best friend. You've got a swimsuit, a pair of shorts, a tank top, and a flirty summer dress on your list of things to buy. The parking lot is crowded, but that's okay; the walk will be nice. You and your friend hop out of the car and skip toward the mall. As you walk into the mall, the air conditioner instantly cools you off and you beeline for your favorite shop. As you cruise the racks, you spot a bikini that you've got to try. Once in the dressing room, you twirl around and love the way you look in it. You feel incredible and can't wait to wear it out. Just then your friend hoists a white sundress over your dressing-room door and says, "I think this will look fabulous on you!" You try it on, and yep, you *do* look fabulous. What other summer clothes do you try on and how great do they look? And more importantly, how will you feel wearing them on the shore?

DATE: _____

EATING PLANNER

This plan will ensure leaner muscle and a higher metabolism.

Breakfast>time_____   Description

○	PROTEIN* (3–5oz/40g)	
○	CARBS (½ cup or 1 slice of bread)	
○	FRUIT (1 cup)	
○	FAT (1 teaspoon)	

Snack>time_____   Description

| ○ | WHEY PROTEIN SHAKE (1 scoop) | |

Jorge recommends Jorge's Packs™ protein drinks. **>** See other recommended snacks at the back of the journal.

Lunch>time_____   Description

○	PROTEIN* (3–5oz/40g)	
○	CARBS (½ cup or 1 slice of bread)	
○	VEGGIES** (2 cups)	
○	FAT (1 teaspoon)	

Snack>time_____   Description

| ○ | WHEY PROTEIN SHAKE (1 scoop) | |

Dinner>time_____   Description

○	PROTEIN* (3–5oz/40g)	
○	VEGGIES** (2–4 cups)	
○	FAT (1 teaspoon)	

Snack>time_____   Description

| ○ | WHEY PROTEIN SHAKE (1 scoop) | |

*If you weigh under 150 pounds, eat 3 ounces of protein at every meal; if you weigh over 150 pounds, eat 5 ounces of protein.

**Veggies = nonstarchy vegetables.

Water (eight 8-oz cups) ○ ○ ○ ○ ○ ○ ○ ○

Multivitamin ○

WORKOUT LOG | WEEK_____OF 8 |

Secondary Workout

DATE_____ DAY_____ OF 56

Start>time_____ Finish>time_____

TOTAL TIME_____

Select weights so that by the end of the fourth rep of each exercise you feel an intensity level of 8.

Muscle Group	Exercise	Weight Used	Intensity Level
CIRCUIT 1			
SHOULDERS			
BICEPS			
TRICEPS			
ABS			

At this point you should be about 6 minutes into your workout.

CIRCUIT 2			
SHOULDERS			
BICEPS			
TRICEPS			
ABS			

At this point you should be about 14 minutes into your workout, including 2 minutes of transition time.

CIRCUIT 3			
SHOULDERS			
BICEPS			
TRICEPS			
ABS			

At this point in your workout you should be at 20 minutes. Congratulations! YOU DID IT!

BONUS CARDIO   26-MINUTE MORNING POWER WALK ○

After my workout I feel_____

(e.g., confident, strong)

< REFLECTIONS >

> > > **There are only two options regarding commitment; you're either in or you're out. There's no such thing as life in-between.**

—PAT RILEY

Day Off! > NO WORKOUT TODAY

REFLECTIONS

_____

_____

_____

_____

Jorge's Meditation > ON-THE-GO: Don't let vacations or business trips stop you from doing your two 12-Second Sequence™ workouts every week. Not only will they give you lots of energy, but you'll also adjust much faster to a new time zone. In addition to your 12-Second Sequence™ moves, take advantage of the local attractions that offer their own unique exercise opportunities, like trails through beautiful parks, bicycle tours, dude ranches, snorkeling, and museum walking tours. Check a travel book or look on the Internet for information before you travel. If you'll be too busy to set aside a block of time for activity, be creative with your time and use every chance you have to be active. Walk wherever you can—around the airport, in-between meetings, or even just around the hotel.

BONUS CARDIO   26-MINUTE MORNING POWER WALK ○

DATE: _____

EATING PLANNER

This plan will ensure leaner muscle and a higher metabolism.

Breakfast>time _____   Description

○	PROTEIN* (3–5oz/40g)	
○	CARBS (½ cup or 1 slice of bread)	
○	FRUIT (1 cup)	
○	FAT (1 teaspoon)	

Snack>time _____   Description

○	WHEY PROTEIN SHAKE (1 scoop)	

Jorge recommends Jorge's Packs™ protein drinks. **>** See other recommended snacks at the back of the journal.

Lunch>time _____   Description

○	PROTEIN* (3–5oz/40g)	
○	CARBS (½ cup or 1 slice of bread)	
○	VEGGIES** (2 cups)	
○	FAT (1 teaspoon)	

Snack>time _____   Description

○	WHEY PROTEIN SHAKE (1 scoop)	

Dinner>time _____   Description

○	PROTEIN* (3–5oz/40g)	
○	VEGGIES** (2–4 cups)	
○	FAT (1 teaspoon)	

Snack>time _____   Description

○	WHEY PROTEIN SHAKE (1 scoop)	

*If you weigh under 150 pounds, eat 3 ounces of protein at every meal; if you weigh over 150 pounds, eat 5 ounces of protein.

**Veggies = nonstarchy vegetables.

Water (eight 8-oz cups) ○ ○ ○ ○ ○ ○ ○ ○

Multivitamin ○

> > > **Whatever the mind can conceive and believe, the mind can achieve.** —NAPOLEON HILL

Day Off! > NO WORKOUT TODAY

REFLECTIONS _____
_____
_____
_____
_____

Jorge's Meditation > **YOUR MOST PRECIOUS GIFT:** Your body is the most precious gift that you have ever been given. Today I'd like you to focus your journal entry on how amazing your body is and why you need to put it first. Remember, you can't take care of anyone else unless you first take care of yourself. Why must you respect and take care of your body? Here are some inspirational thoughts to get you started; repeat them out loud and then write your own in your journal: "I have only one body. I cannot get another one if I ruin this one. My body is the only real instrument to live my life's purpose. My body is my vehicle to being an active parent. My eyes allow me to see the beautiful smile of my lover's face. My ears allow me to hear the relaxing sound of the ocean waves. My arms allow me to hug and show my love for my friends, family, and kids. My legs allow me to dance, play, and travel this world." Take care of this amazing gift you've worked so hard to improve over the past eight weeks.

BONUS CARDIO 26-MINUTE MORNING POWER WALK ○

DATE:

EATING PLANNER

This plan will ensure leaner muscle and a higher metabolism.

Breakfast>time_____

Description

○	PROTEIN* (3–5oz/40g)	
○	CARBS (½ cup or 1 slice of bread)	
○	FRUIT (1 cup)	
○	FAT (1 teaspoon)	

Snack>time_____

Description

○	WHEY PROTEIN SHAKE (1 scoop)	

Jorge recommends Jorge's Packs™ protein drinks. **>** See other recommended snacks at the back of the journal.

Lunch>time_____

Description

○	PROTEIN* (3–5oz/40g)	
○	CARBS (½ cup or 1 slice of bread)	
○	VEGGIES** (2 cups)	
○	FAT (1 teaspoon)	

Snack>time_____

Description

○	WHEY PROTEIN SHAKE (1 scoop)	

Dinner>time_____

Description

○	PROTEIN* (3–5oz/40g)	
○	VEGGIES** (2–4 cups)	
○	FAT (1 teaspoon)	

Snack>time_____

Description

○	WHEY PROTEIN SHAKE (1 scoop)	

*If you weigh under 150 pounds, eat 3 ounces of protein at every meal; if you weigh over 150 pounds, eat 5 ounces of protein.

**Veggies = nonstarchy vegetables.

Water (eight 8-oz cups) ○ ○ ○ ○ ○ ○ ○ ○

Multivitamin ○

> > > **Shoot for the moon. Even if you miss, you'll land among the stars.**

—LES BROWN

Day Off! > NO WORKOUT TODAY

REFLECTIONS

_____

_____

_____

_____

Jorge's Meditation > CONGRATULATIONS!: You did it! You've successfully completed your 12-Second Sequence™ 8-Week Challenge! By now you should be able to see those long, lean muscles you've been working so hard to shape and tone. You have lost fat so your clothes fit better and you look more defined. Regardless of how much weight you've lost, you FINISHED this challenge—and that's what really matters. Your commitment to the 8-Week Challenge and the effort you put into each exercise will affect other areas of your life as well. You might start getting up earlier in the morning to work out, and you'll probably lose interest in eating unhealthy foods. Even more inspiring, your commitment to improving your health may motivate someone else to take control of her life and fitness. You could even become a mentor! Share what you've learned about fitness and the skills you developed with someone who wants to improve his own health. You might just change someone's life!

BONUS CARDIO 26-MINUTE MORNING POWER WALK ○

DATE:

EATING PLANNER

This plan will ensure leaner muscle and a higher metabolism.

Breakfast>time_____   Description

○	PROTEIN* (3–5oz/40g)	
○	CARBS (½ cup or 1 slice of bread)	
○	FRUIT (1 cup)	
○	FAT (1 teaspoon)	

Snack>time_____   Description

○	WHEY PROTEIN SHAKE (1 scoop)	

Jorge recommends Jorge's Packs™ protein drinks. **>** See other recommended snacks at the back of the journal.

Lunch>time_____   Description

○	PROTEIN* (3–5oz/40g)	
○	CARBS (½ cup or 1 slice of bread)	
○	VEGGIES** (2 cups)	
○	FAT (1 teaspoon)	

Snack>time_____   Description

○	WHEY PROTEIN SHAKE (1 scoop)	

Dinner>time_____   Description

○	PROTEIN* (3–5oz/40g)	
○	VEGGIES** (2–4 cups)	
○	FAT (1 teaspoon)	

Snack>time_____   Description

○	WHEY PROTEIN SHAKE (1 scoop)	

*If you weigh under 150 pounds, eat 3 ounces of protein at every meal; if you weigh over 150 pounds, eat 5 ounces of protein.

**Veggies = nonstarchy vegetables.

Water (eight 8-oz cups) ○ ○ ○ ○ ○ ○ ○ ○

Multivitamin ○

< FUTURE GOALS >

SUCCESS!

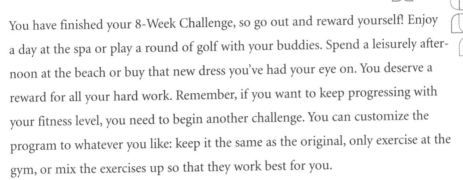

You have finished your 8-Week Challenge, so go out and reward yourself! Enjoy a day at the spa or play a round of golf with your buddies. Spend a leisurely afternoon at the beach or buy that new dress you've had your eye on. You deserve a reward for all your hard work. Remember, if you want to keep progressing with your fitness level, you need to begin another challenge. You can customize the program to whatever you like: keep it the same as the original, only exercise at the gym, or mix the exercises up so that they work best for you.

I'm so proud of you for completing this 8-Week Challenge. Congratulations and good luck!

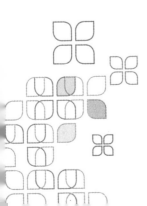

PROTEIN

(3 ounces if you weigh less than 150 pounds;
5 ounces if you weigh more than 150 pounds)

- 95% lean beef
- beef tenderloin
- chicken/turkey breast (skinless)
- eggs (whole)
- fish
- lamb
- London broil
- low-fat cottage cheese
- ostrich
- pork tenderloin
- round steak
- shellfish

CARBOHYDRATE

(½ cup or 1 slice of bread)

- brown rice
- buckwheat
- oatmeal
- sweet potatoes
- wheat germ
- whole grain flour
- whole grain cereal
- whole wheat bread
- whole wheat pasta
- whole wheat tortilla
- wild rice

VEGETABLES (NONSTARCHY)

(2 to 4 cups)

- alfalfa sprouts
- asparagus
- beets (minimize)
- bell peppers
- broccoli
- Brussels sprouts
- cabbage
- cauliflower
- celery
- chiles
- cucumber
- eggplant (minimize)
- garlic
- green beans
- green onions
- lettuce
- mushrooms
- parsnips (minimize)
- radishes
- spinach
- squash
- tomatoes
- turnips (minimize)
- watercress
- zucchini

FATS

(1 teaspoon)

- almonds (6)
- almond butter
- avocado (⅛)
- cashews (6)
- flaxseed oil
- olive oil
- peanut butter
- peanuts (10)

FRUITS
(1 item or 2 cups diced)

- apples
- blackberries
- blueberries
- grapefruit
- grapes
- lemons
- limes
- melons
- peaches
- pears
- strawberries

SNACKS
(3 per day)

- Jorge's Packs™ Whey Protein Shake
- low-fat cottage cheese (½ cup)
- 1 ounce beef jerky
- ½ cup chopped cooked chicken breast meat
- 3 ounces tuna or salmon (canned or pouch)
- 6 ounces plain nonfat yogurt

FREEBIES

- water
- Propel® Fit Water™
- club soda
- mineral water
- coffee (minimize)
- diet soda (minimize)

SUGAR SUBSTITUTES
(in moderation)

- Stevia
- Splenda®

SWEETS
(in moderation)

- sugar-free candies
- sugar-free gum
- sugar-free gelatin desserts

FLAVOR ENHANCERS

- low-sodium broth
- garlic
- herbs (fresh or dried)
- lemon or lime juice
- mustard
- pickles
- salsa
- spices
- low-sodium soy sauce
- vinegar
- Worcestershire sauce

SUPPLEMENTS
(use daily)

- Barlean's flax oil
- Jorge's Packs™ Vitamins
- multivitamin

Breakfast

FAST FOOD

Subway® Western Egg with Cheese Breakfast Sandwich (1)
Add a piece of fruit.

McDonald's® Egg McMuffin® (1)
Add a piece of fruit.

Denny's® Veggie Cheese Omelet with Egg Beaters® (1)
Add a piece of fruit.

FROZEN FOOD

Weight Watchers® Smart Ones® English Muffin Sandwich (1)
Add a whey protein shake and a piece of fruit.

Lean Pockets® Bacon, Egg, and Cheese (1)
Add a whey protein shake and a piece of fruit.

Lean Pockets® Sausage, Egg, and Cheese (1)
Add a whey protein shake and a piece of fruit.

Lunch

FAST FOOD

Arby's® Santa Fe Salad with Grilled Chicken (1)
Add one serving of light buttermilk ranch dressing.

Baja Fresh® Shrimp Tacos (2)
Add a side salad (2 cups) and a squeeze of lemon for dressing.

Blimpie® Turkey Sub, 6-inch, on wheat (1)

Burger King® TenderGrill® Chicken Filet Salad (1)
Add one serving of Ken's® Fat-Free Ranch Dressing.

Chick-fil-A® Chicken Cool Wrap® (1)
Add a side salad (2 cups) and a squeeze of lemon for dressing.

Chick-fil-A® Southwest Chargrilled Chicken Salad (1)
Add a squeeze of lemon for dressing, half a packet of Garlic and Butter Croutons, and a small order of Hearty Breast of Chicken Soup.

Chipotle Bowl with Barbacoa (1)
Ask for double lettuce, fajita vegetables, red tomatillo salsa, and black beans. No rice.

Dairy Queen® Grilled Chicken Sandwich (1)
Add a side salad with one serving of fat-free Italian dressing.

KFC® Tender Roast® Sandwich Without Sauce (1)
Ask for an additional 2 ounces of grilled chicken and add a house side salad with Hidden Valley® Golden Italian Light Ranch Dressing.

McDonald's® Asian Salad with Grilled Chicken
Ask for an additional 1 ounce of chicken and a side of Butter Garlic Croutons. Add a squeeze of lemon for dressing.

Rubio's Fresh Mexican Grill® Mahi Mahi Taco (1)
Ask for an additional 3 ounces of mahimahi and add a side salad (2 cups) with 2 tablespoons salsa for dressing.

Rubio's Fresh Mexican Grill® Carne Asada Street Tacos (2)
Ask for an additional 2 ounces of carne asada and add half a side order of pinto beans and a side salad (2 cups) with 2 tablespoons salsa as dressing.

Rubio's Fresh Mexican Grill® HealthMex® Chicken Taco (2)
Ask for an additional 1 ounce of chicken and add a side salad (2 cups) with 2 tablespoons salsa as dressing.

Subway® Club Sandwich, 6-inch, on whole wheat (1)
Add a Veggie Delite salad with fat-free Italian dressing.

FROZEN FOOD

Lean Cuisine® Café Classics Chicken à L'Orange (1)
Add a mixed green salad (2 cups) with a squeeze of lemon and 1 teaspoon flaxseed oil for dressing.

Lean Cuisine® Casual Eating Classics™ Roasted Garlic Chicken Pizza (1)
Add a mixed green salad (2 cups) with a squeeze of lemon and 1 teaspoon flaxseed oil for dressing.

Lean Cuisine® One Dish Favorites™ Classic Five Cheese Lasagna (1)
Add a mixed green salad (2 cups) with a squeeze of lemon and 1 teaspoon flaxseed oil for dressing.

Healthy Choice® Flavor Adventures Chicken Tuscany (1)
Add a mixed green salad (2 cups) with a squeeze of lemon and 1 teaspoon flaxseed oil for dressing.

Healthy Choice® Flavor Adventures Grilled Whiskey Steak (1)
Add a mixed green salad (2 cups) with a squeeze of lemon and 1 teaspoon flaxseed oil for dressing.

Dinner
FAST FOOD

Chipotle Bowl with Chicken (1)
Ask for double lettuce, fajita vegetables, green tomatillo salsa, and tomato salsa. No rice or beans.

Daphne's® Greek Chicken Salad (1)
Ask for no pita and extra salad. Add a squeeze of lemon for dressing.

KFC® Roasted Caesar Salad (1)
Ask for an additional 3 ounces of roasted chicken and Hidden Valley® Light Golden Ranch Dressing.

McDonald's® Bacon Ranch Salad with Grilled Chicken (1)
Ask for an additional 2 ounces of grilled chicken and Newman's Own® Low-Fat Balsamic Vinaigrette.

Subway® Grilled Chicken Breast and Spinach Salad (1)
Ask for an additional 3 ounces of grilled chicken and fat-free Italian dressing.

FROZEN FOOD

Gorton's® Cajun Blackened Grilled Fillets (3)
Add a mixed green salad (3 cups) with lemon juice and 1 teaspoon flaxseed oil for dressing.

Gorton's® Shrimp Temptations Scampi (2 servings)
Add a mixed green salad (3 cups) with lemon juice and 1 teaspoon flaxseed oil for dressing.

Tyson® Mesquite Breast Fillets (Bagged) (2)
Add a mixed green salad (3 cups) with lemon juice and 1 teaspoon flaxseed oil for dressing.

Go to 12second.com for more fast/frozen food ideas.

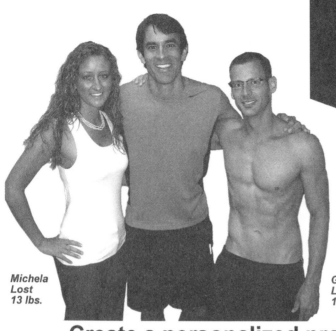

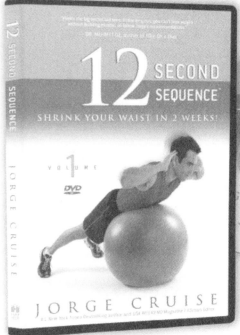
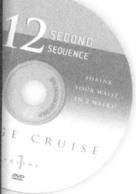

The 12-Second Sequence™ Hardcover

The 12-Second Sequence™ is fitness superstar Jorge Cruise's newest revolutionary method of resistance training that burns fat, shrinks your waistline, and gets you into the best shape of your life—and all it takes is two twenty-minute workouts each week. Based on the latest groundbreaking research in exercise physiology, the 12-Second Sequence™ proves that the key to success is not in exercising *more*, but in exercising *smarter*. Available everywhere books are sold.

The 12-Second Sequence™ Audiobook

Jorge takes you through the science and theory behind The 12-Second Sequence™ in this audio recording that makes it easy for you to understand the principles outlined in the core book. This CD is the perfect solution for beginners or people who just don't have the time to read the core book. Available everywhere books are sold.

The 12-Second Sequence™ (Spanish edition)

Do you know a Spanish-speaker who needs to get in shape? The Spanish edition of *The 12-Second Sequence*™ is the perfect gift for a friend who wants to get fit, eat smart, and achieve his or her ideal body. Available everywhere books are sold.